The Homemade Apothecary

Maggie Damien, PhD

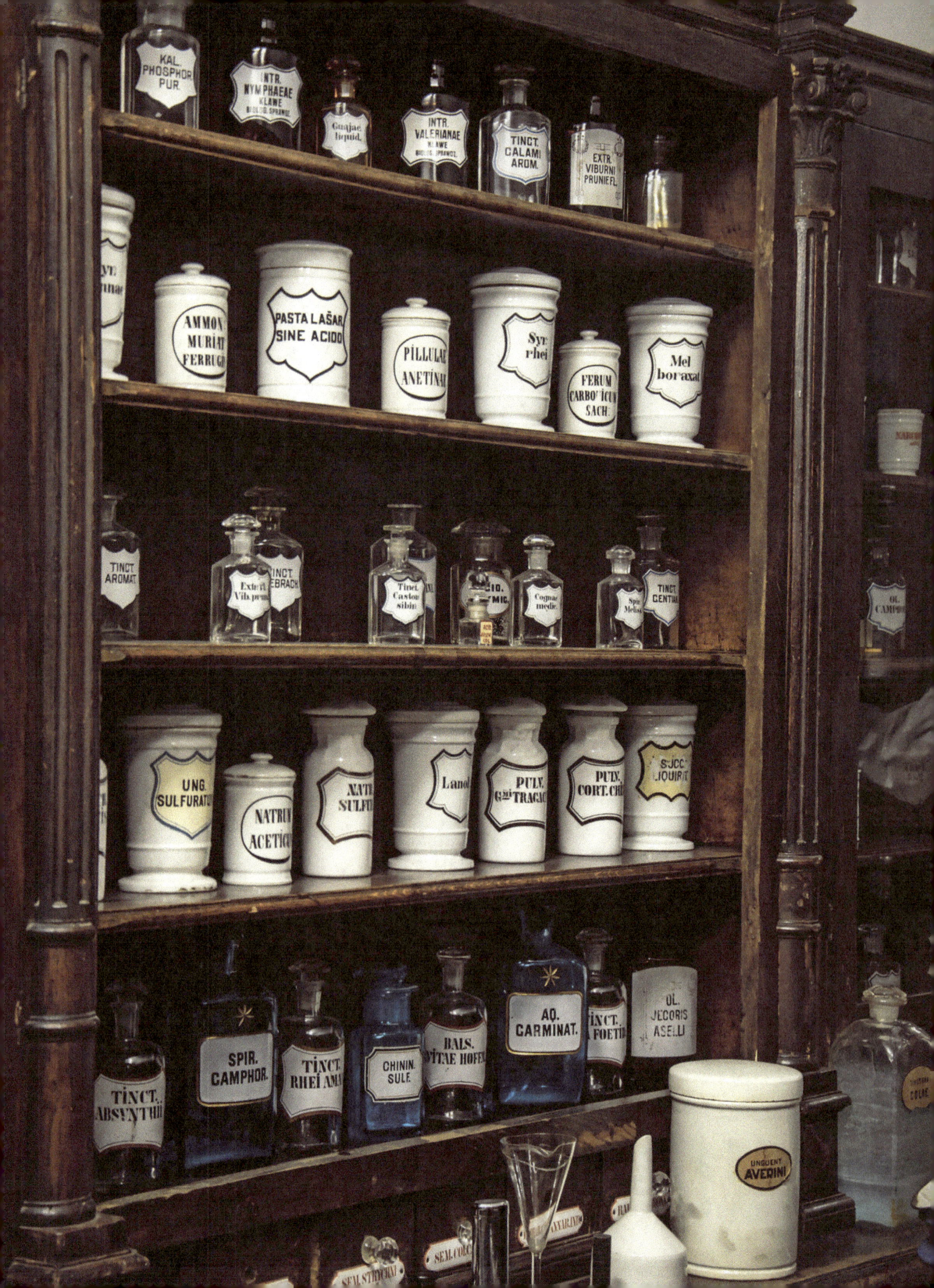

Table of Contents

Part 1: The World of Home Apothecary
1. Introduction to Herbal Medicine Across Cultures
   - The Global Heritage of Healing with Herbs
   - How Traditional Practices Inform Modern Remedies
2. Essential Tools and Ingredients
   - Universal Equipment for Herbal Preparation
   - Unique Regional Ingredients and Their Applications
3. Understanding Herbal Medicine
   - Active Plant Compounds and Their Benefits
   - The Science of Healing Plants

Part 2: The Global Herbal Repository
1. African Herbal Traditions
   - Key Herbs and Their Uses:
     - Moringa (Nutrient Boost)
     - Baobab (Immunity and Digestive Health)
     - Devil's Claw (Joint Pain Relief)
     - Hibiscus (Blood Pressure Regulation)
     - Neem (Antiviral and Antibacterial Properties)
   - Indigenous Herbal Practices
2. Asian Herbal Traditions
   - Chinese, Indian (Ayurvedic), and Southeast Asian Contributions
   - Key Herbs and Their Uses:
     - Ginseng (Vitality and Energy)
     - Turmeric (Anti-Inflammatory)
     - Gotu Kola (Cognitive Health)
     - Licorice Root (Digestive Aid)
     - Holy Basil (Tulsi) (Stress Relief)

1. European Herbal Traditions
   - From Ancient Rome to Modern Herbalism
   - Key Herbs and Their Uses:
     - Lavender (Relaxation and Skin Care)
     - Chamomile (Sleep Aid and Digestive Soother)
     - Elderberry (Immune Support)
     - St. John's Wort (Mood Enhancement)
     - Thyme (Antiseptic and Respiratory Health)
2. Native American Herbal Traditions
   - Sacred Plants of Indigenous Cultures
   - Key Herbs and Their Uses:
     - Echinacea (Immune Booster)
     - Sage (Cleansing and Respiratory Aid)
     - Black Cohosh (Women's Health)
     - Willow Bark (Pain Relief)
     - Yarrow (Wound Healing)
3. Latin American Herbal Traditions
   - Healing Practices from the Amazon and Beyond
   - Key Herbs and Their Uses:
     - Chanca Piedra (Kidney Health)
     - Guarana (Energy Boost)
     - Yerba Mate (Cognitive Stimulant)
     - Achiote (Annatto) (Anti-Inflammatory)
     - Quinine (Malaria Treatment)
4. Oceanic and Polynesian Herbal Traditions
   - Healing Practices of Island Cultures
   - Key Herbs and Their Uses:
     - Kava (Stress and Anxiety Relief)
     - Noni (Immunity and Skin Health)
     - Breadfruit Leaves (Diabetes Support)

Part 3: Crafting Herbal Remedies
1. Basic Preparations for Beginners
    - Teas, Infusions, and Decoctions
    - Tinctures, Oils, and Salves
2. Advanced Techniques
    - Making Herbal Capsules and Powders
    - Crafting Herbal Ferments and Tonics
3. Integrating Aromatherapy
    - Essential Oils from Every Continent
    - Blending for Health and Wellness

Part 4: Remedies for Every Need
1. Building Your Herbal First Aid Kit
    - Remedies for Cuts, Bruises, and Infections
2. Remedies for Common Ailments
    - Immune Support (Colds, Flu, Allergies)
    - Digestive Health (Bloating, Nausea, Constipation)
    - Stress and Anxiety Relief
    - Skin Health
3. Herbal Support for Women's Health
    - Menstrual Health, Fertility, and Menopause
4. Herbs for Men's Wellness
    - Energy, Stamina, and Prostate Health
5. Herbs for Children
    - Gentle Remedies for Childhood Illnesses
6. Eldercare with Herbs
    - Cognitive Support and Chronic Pain Relief

Part 5: Global Herbal Wisdom
1. The African Apothecary
    - Foraging and Growing African Herbs
2. The Asian Apothecary
    - Principles of Traditional Chinese Medicine and Ayurveda
3. The European Apothecary
    - Combining Ancient and Modern Herbal Wisdom
4. The Americas' Apothecary

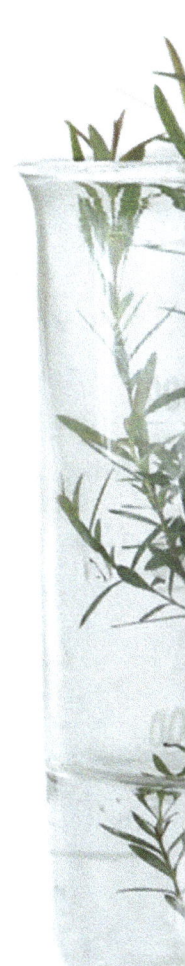

- Sacred Healing Practices from Indigenous Communities
1. The Island Apothecary
    - Polynesian and Oceanic Healing Secrets

Part 6: Practical Applications
1. Herbal Beauty and Self-Care
    - Skin and Hair Care Recipes
2. Herbal Nutrition
    - Cooking with Medicinal Herbs: Global Recipes
3. Seasonal Wellness with Herbs
    - Preparing for Flu Season, Allergy Season, and More

Part 7: Sustaining Your Apothecary
1. Herb Gardening Across Climates
    - Growing African, Asian, and European Herbs at Home
2. Foraging and Ethical Harvesting
    - How to Harvest Herbs Responsibly
3. Storing and Maintaining Your Remedies
    - Extending the Shelf Life of Herbal Products

Part 8: Resources and References
1. Glossary of Herbs and Active Compounds
2. Index of Remedies by Ailment
3. Suggested Further Reading and Courses
4. Acknowledgments

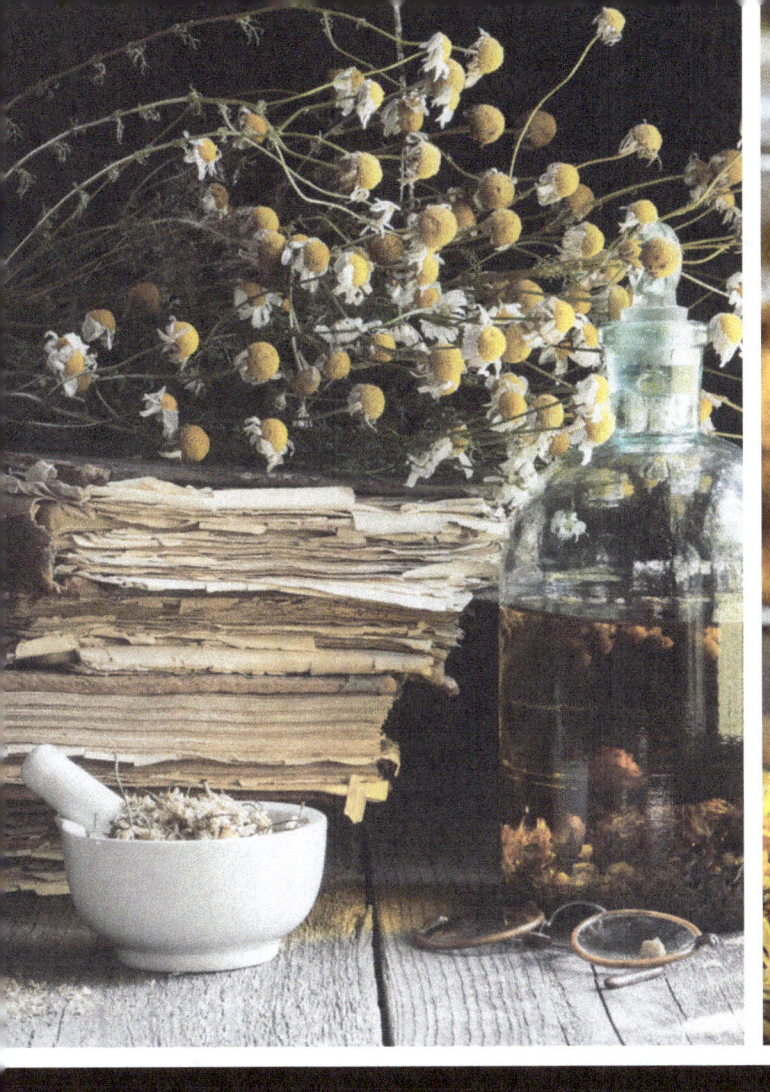
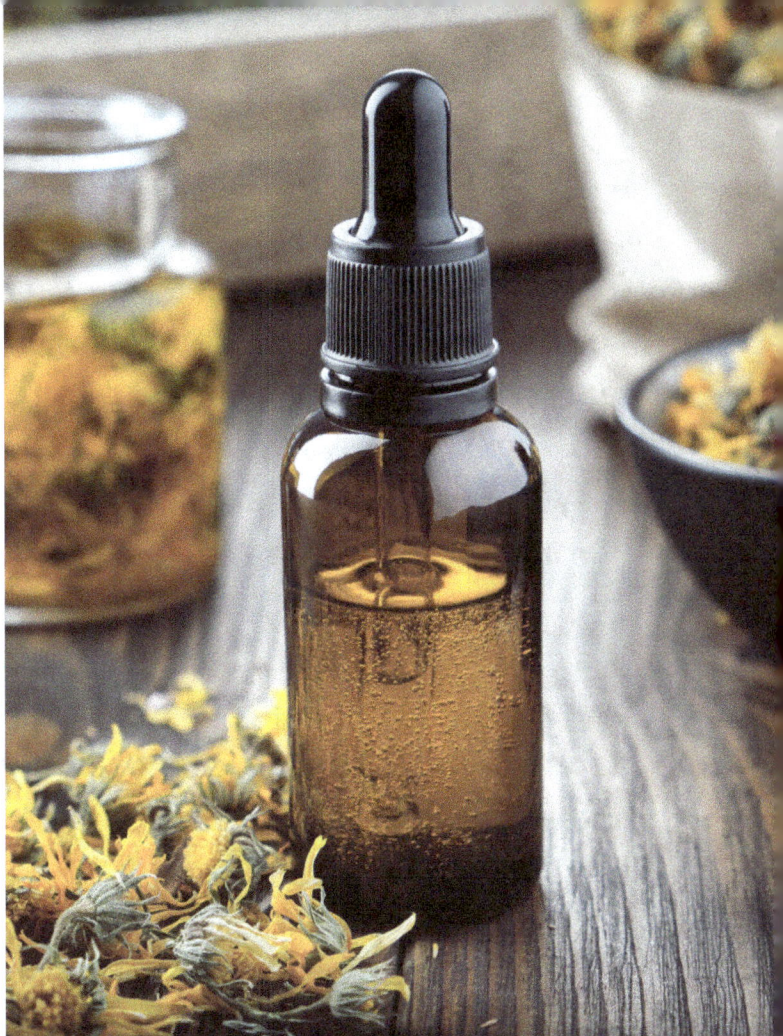

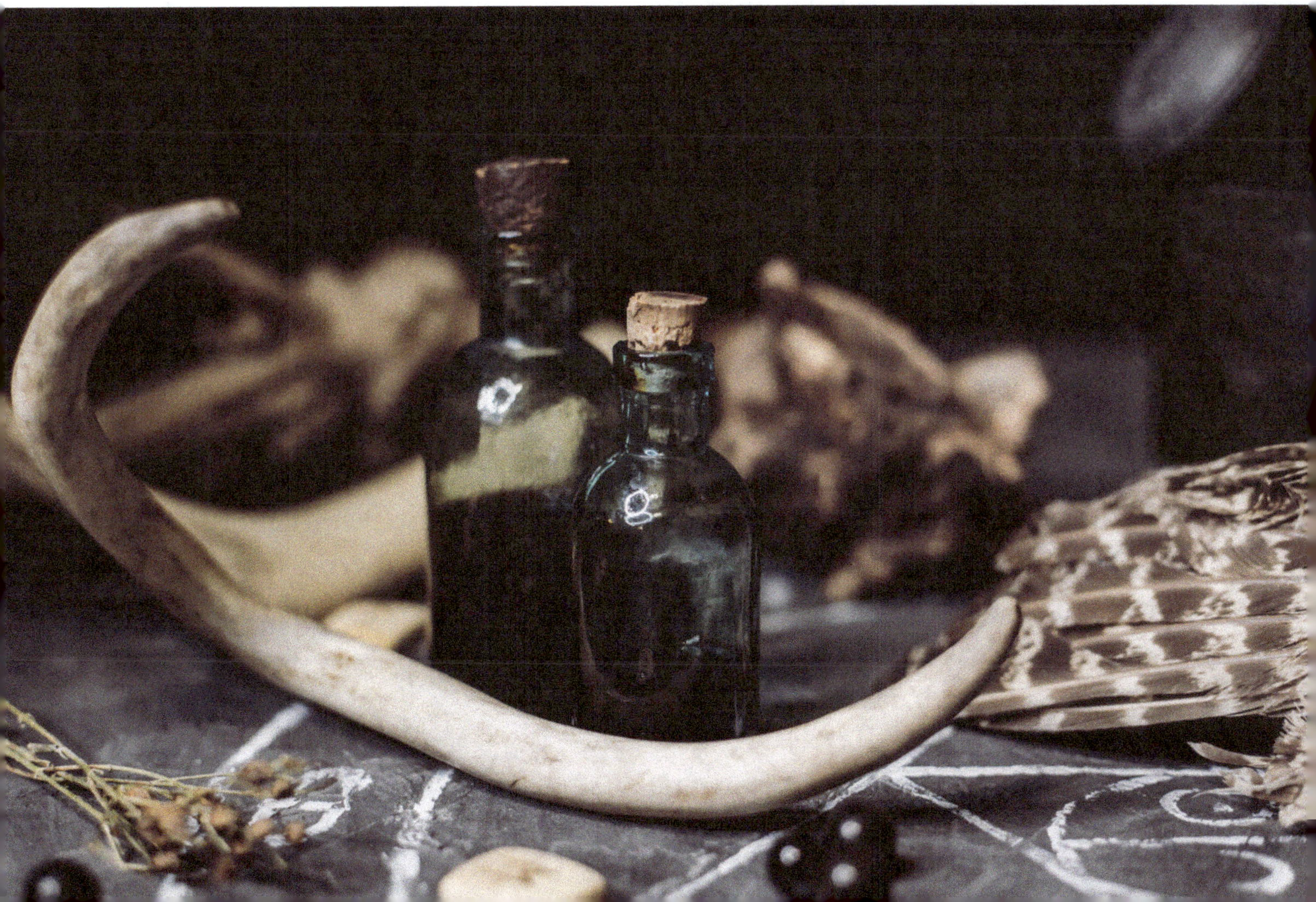

Customer Experinences

I have struggled with erectile dysfunction for years, trying various treatments with little success. After reading The Homemade Apothecary, I found the section on men's wellness and started using remedies with ginseng and maca root. The results have been incredible, and I feel like myself again. The detailed pictures of the herbs made it easy to recognize what I needed."
— Jonathan M., Dallas, Texas

"As a first-time mom, I experienced severe morning sickness during my pregnancy. The chapter on women's health led me to ginger and peppermint remedies, and within days, I felt relief. The vibrant photos helped me trust that I was using the right ingredients."
— Emily R., UK

My hair was thinning badly, and I had tried countless products. When I read about African herbs like moringa and neem in this book, I made the recommended hair mask. My hair looks thicker and healthier now. The pictures of the herbs were so detailed, I could easily spot them at the local market."
— Samantha T., Los Angeles, California

"Seasonal allergies have always been a nightmare for me. After reading The Homemade Apothecary, I made a tea with nettle and elderflower as suggested. The relief was almost instant. Seeing the high-quality images of these herbs gave me confidence to forage responsibly."
— David H., CA

"I've dealt with severe digestive issues for years, including bloating and constipation. The chapter on digestive health introduced me to turmeric and fennel seed remedies. Within a week of use, my symptoms improved drastically. I loved the clear pictures of each herb—it made shopping so much easier!"
— Caroline B., Atlanta, Georgia

"My son often gets colds during winter, and I hated relying on over-the-counter medicine. This book's section on immune support guided me to echinacea and elderberry syrup recipes. He hasn't caught a cold in months! The photographs of the herbs are stunning and so helpful."
— Hannah W., Amsterdam

"Chronic pain in my joints was affecting my mobility. Thanks to the book's insights on devil's claw and turmeric, I've found a natural remedy that works better than painkillers. The step-by-step instructions paired with herb images made everything easy to follow."
— Richard P., Phoenix, Arizona

"I've had insomnia for years, but the chamomile and lavender remedies in this book have changed my life. The pictures of these herbs inspired me to grow them in my garden, and now I enjoy restful sleep naturally."
— Eleanor F., Leeds, UK

"Battling anxiety was overwhelming, but the section on stress relief introduced me to holy basil (tulsi) tea. The calming effect was immediate, and I feel much more centered. The vivid herb photos were incredibly helpful in identifying tulsi at my local store."
— James K., Germany

"After a nasty burn in the kitchen, I turned to the book's first aid section. The aloe vera remedy worked wonders for my skin. The detailed photos of aloe and other first-aid plants are like having a herbalist by my side."
— Linda J., London

"My daughter's eczema made her skin itchy and red. Following this book's recipes using calendula and coconut oil brought her relief within days. The images of calendula flowers are gorgeous and made finding the right herb easy."
— Megan S., Miami, Florida

"I used to get frequent migraines, and nothing seemed to work. After discovering feverfew in The Homemade Apothecary, I started drinking the recommended tea, and my headaches have almost disappeared. The herb photos in the book made it easy to identify feverfew in my garden."
— Andrew L., Edinburgh.

Preface

Herbs have always held a unique place in human history. Long before the advent of modern medicine, our ancestors turned to the earth for healing, wisdom, and nourishment. Every culture, from the bustling markets of Marrakech to the serene landscapes of Kyoto, has cultivated a deep relationship with medicinal plants. Today, as more people seek natural remedies to complement conventional medicine, the power of herbs is being rediscovered and celebrated.

The Homemade Apothecary was born from my passion for this timeless connection between humans and the healing properties of plants. Over the years, I've worked closely with herbalists, scientists, and indigenous communities to unravel the stories behind some of the world's most potent remedies. This book is my attempt to bring that wealth of knowledge into your hands, in a format that is both accessible and deeply rooted in tradition.

I envisioned this book as more than a guide—it's a journey across cultures, climates, and centuries. Whether you're a beginner curious about herbal teas or an experienced practitioner looking to expand your knowledge of global remedies, The Homemade Apothecary offers something for everyone. It provides practical techniques for crafting herbal solutions, detailed profiles of key herbs from every corner of the world, and insights into how these plants can enhance your health and well-being.

As you explore the pages of this book, you'll also notice a focus on ethical foraging and sustainability. Herbs are gifts from the earth, and it is our responsibility to use them mindfully. By cultivating, harvesting, and preparing remedies responsibly, we ensure that these resources remain available for generations to come.

This book is a labor of love, drawn from years of study, travel, and personal practice. My hope is that it will inspire you to embrace the healing potential of herbs and deepen your connection to nature. May it empower you to build your own apothecary at home—a space where the magic of plants meets the art of healing.

With gratitude,

Maggie Damien, PhD

About the Author

Dr. Maggie Damien is an internationally renowned herbalist, researcher, and educator with over two decades of experience in traditional and modern herbal medicine. A PhD holder in Ethnobotany, she has devoted her career to exploring the medicinal properties of plants and their applications across diverse cultures. Her passion for natural healing began in her childhood, growing up in a family that valued nature's remedies, sparking a lifelong dedication to uncovering the secrets of plants.

Dr. Damien has traveled extensively across Africa, Asia, Europe, and the Americas, collaborating with indigenous communities to document their herbal traditions. Her work bridges ancient wisdom and modern science, ensuring that age-old practices are preserved while being adapted for contemporary use. She has published numerous academic papers on herbal pharmacology and has been a keynote speaker at global conferences on sustainable herbal practices.

In The Homemade Apothecary, Dr. Damien combines her scholarly expertise with a heartfelt commitment to empowering individuals to take charge of their health. Her engaging writing style and practical approach make this book a must-have for anyone interested in herbal medicine.

When she's not immersed in her research, Dr. Damien enjoys tending to her herb garden and teaching workshops on holistic wellness. She lives in the scenic countryside of Vermont with her husband, two children, and a playful golden retriever named Basil.

Foreword

As someone who has dedicated much of my life to the study and practice of herbal medicine, I can confidently say that The Homemade Apothecary is a groundbreaking contribution to the field. Dr. Maggie Damien's ability to bridge ancient traditions with modern science is nothing short of remarkable.

In a world where pharmaceuticals dominate the conversation around health, we often forget the immense power of plants. For centuries, herbs have been humanity's first line of defense against illness, offering solutions for ailments ranging from minor colds to chronic conditions. What sets this book apart is its global perspective, inviting readers to explore how cultures across the world use herbs in their daily lives.

Dr. Damien's meticulous research and attention to detail shine through on every page. Whether she's detailing the anti-inflammatory properties of turmeric from India, the immune-boosting benefits of echinacea used by Native Americans, or the stress-relieving qualities of kava from Polynesia, she brings each herb to life with vivid descriptions and practical applications.

Equally impressive is her commitment to sustainability and ethical practices. At a time when overharvesting threatens some of the planet's most valuable medicinal plants, this book serves as a call to action for responsible stewardship. Dr. Damien not only teaches us how to use herbs but also how to respect the ecosystems that provide them.

Reading The Homemade Apothecary feels like embarking on a journey through time and across continents, guided by an expert who understands both the science and the soul of herbal medicine. Whether you are looking to address specific health concerns, enhance your well-being, or simply learn about the wonders of the plant kingdom, this book will become an invaluable resource in your library.

Reading The Homemade Apothecary feels like embarking on a journey through time and across continents, guided by an expert who understands both the science and the soul of herbal medicine. Whether you are looking to address specific health concerns, enhance your well-being, or simply learn about the wonders of the plant kingdom, this book will become an invaluable resource in your library.

Dr. Damien's work is a testament to the enduring power of herbal medicine and its ability to transform lives. I am honored to introduce this remarkable book and encourage readers to embrace the wisdom it offers.

Sincerely,

Dr. James S,

Herbal Medicine Specialist, Speaker, and Author

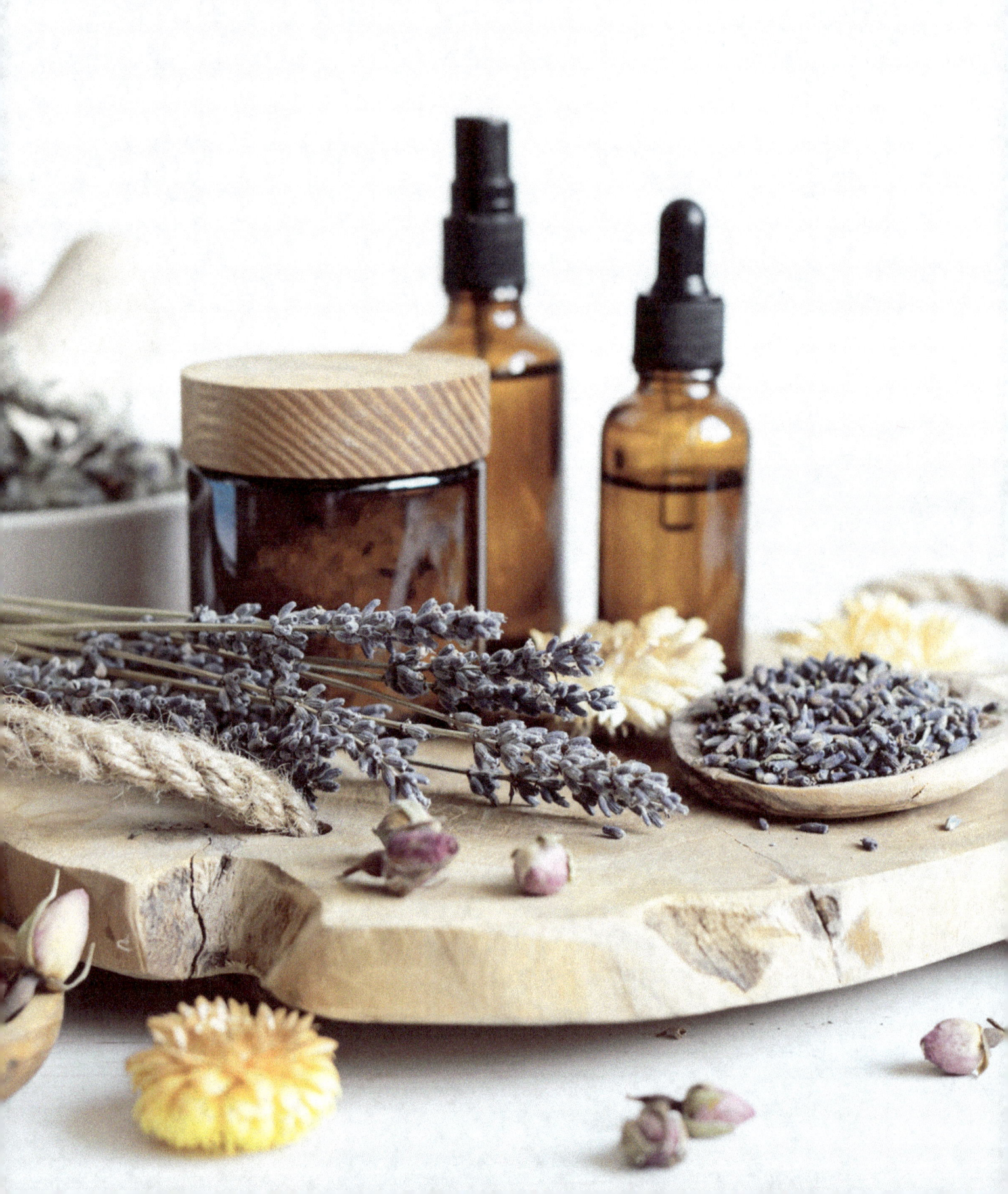

Introduction to Herbal Medicine Across Cultures

Herbal medicine, often called the "people's medicine," has roots as deep as human civilization itself. Across every corner of the globe, societies have relied on plants to cure ailments, enhance health, and preserve vitality. From the dense forests of the Amazon to the arid savannas of Africa, and the rich spice markets of Asia to the meadows of Europe, the wisdom of nature's pharmacy has shaped cultural identities and health practices.

The Global Heritage of Healing with Herbs

The use of herbs for medicinal purposes predates written history, with archaeological evidence revealing that plants have been used for healing for tens of thousands of years. Each culture contributed unique knowledge, driven by its environment, spirituality, and cultural practices.

1. African Healing TraditionsAfrica is home to some of the oldest herbal medicine systems, with an emphasis on holistic care and the interconnectedness of body, mind, and spirit. The practices of traditional healers, such as Sangomas in Southern Africa, rely on plants like baobab, moringa, and devil's claw for treating a range of conditions. These remedies are often accompanied by rituals and community practices, reflecting the deeply spiritual aspect of African healing traditions.
2. Asian Herbal Systems
    - Traditional Chinese Medicine (TCM): Over 3,000 years old, TCM emphasizes balance, particularly through the concepts of yin and yang. Plants like ginseng, gingko biloba, and reishi mushrooms are staples in addressing energy imbalances, boosting immunity, and supporting longevity.
    - Ayurveda from India: A holistic system, Ayurveda uses herbs like turmeric, ashwagandha, and tulsi to balance the body's doshas (Vata, Pitta, and Kapha). It integrates diet, lifestyle, and herbal therapies in promoting health.

- Southeast Asian Practices: Regions like Indonesia and Thailand contribute with remedies like lemongrass, galangal, and non-timber forest herbs, used in tonics, compresses, and teas for detoxification and vitality.

3. European Herbalism: European herbal medicine was significantly influenced by Greek, Roman, and medieval practices. Notable figures like Hippocrates and Galen laid the groundwork for Western medicine, emphasizing the importance of plants like thyme, sage, and rosemary. The Middle Ages saw monasteries become repositories of herbal knowledge, while the Renaissance rekindled scientific interest in medicinal plants, paving the way for modern pharmacology.

4. Indigenous Practices of the Americas: Native American tribes have long used plants like echinacea, black cohosh, and willow bark. Their approach blends physical and spiritual healing, often performed in the context of ceremonies. The Amazon's biodiversity has also provided countless remedies, such as cat's claw and chanca piedra, known for their antiviral and anti-inflammatory properties.

5. Oceanic and Polynesian Traditions: Island cultures, such as those in Polynesia, incorporate plants like kava and noni for mental health and immune support. The apothecary of the islands highlights sustainable practices, respecting the limited natural resources of these regions.

How Traditional Practices Inform Modern Remedies

While traditional medicine was often dismissed during the rise of Western biomedicine, its contributions to modern pharmacology are undeniable. Many of today's most vital medications are derived from plants initially used in traditional practices.

1. **Pharmacological Advancements**
   - **Willow Bark to Aspirin:** Native American and European herbalists used willow bark for pain relief, leading to the development of aspirin.
   - **Cinchona Bark to Quinine:** South American traditional medicine inspired the use of quinine to treat malaria.
   - **Rosy Periwinkle to Cancer Treatment:** This Madagascar-native plant led to the discovery of vincristine and vinblastine, drugs used in cancer therapy.

1. **Integrative Medicine**
2. Modern medicine increasingly incorporates traditional practices, recognizing their value in treating chronic conditions, improving quality of life, and managing stress. Herbal supplements like *turmeric* for inflammation, *ginseng* for energy, and *peppermint* for digestion are examples of this integration.
3. **Scientific Validation**
4. With the rise of evidence-based approaches, herbs used in traditional practices are subjected to rigorous scientific studies. Compounds like curcumin from turmeric and silymarin from milk thistle have been validated for their therapeutic benefits, bridging the gap between ancient wisdom and modern science.
5. **Sustainability and Ethical Harvesting**

Herbal medicine is a living bridge between the past and the present, uniting cultural wisdom and scientific discovery. It serves not only as a reminder of humanity's deep connection with nature but also as a testament to the ingenuity of cultures worldwide in using plants to promote health and well-being. As we embrace the global heritage of herbal medicine, we also recognize its potential to inspire a future where traditional and modern practices coexist harmoniously, advancing human health in sustainable and inclusive ways.

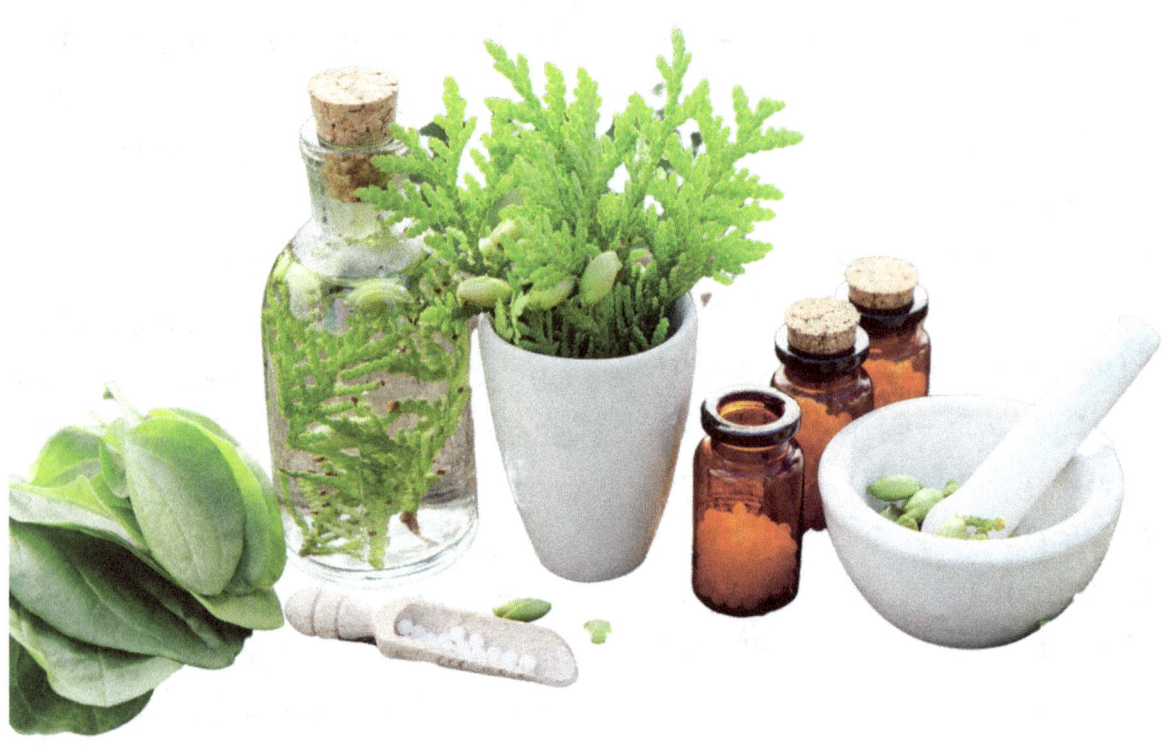

Essential Tools and Ingredients

Preparing herbal remedies requires specific tools and ingredients to maximize the therapeutic potential of plants. Whether you're a beginner or an experienced herbalist, understanding the universal equipment and unique regional ingredients is vital to creating effective and safe preparations.

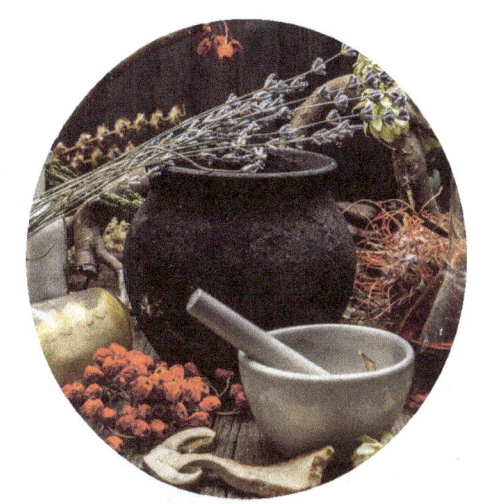

Universal Equipment for Herbal Preparation

The tools used in herbal preparation are simple yet essential for processing, storing, and using herbs effectively. Here are the key categories of equipment:

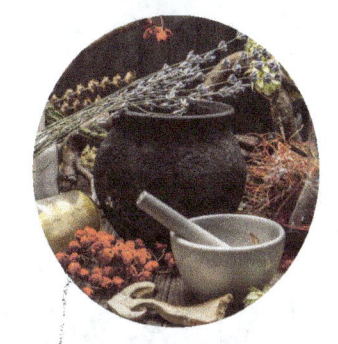

1. Harvesting Tools
    - Shears and Scissors: For cleanly cutting herbs without damaging the plant.
    - Gloves: To protect hands when handling potentially irritating or toxic plants.
    - Baskets or Cloth Bags: Ideal for collecting herbs while preserving their freshness.
2. Drying and Storage Equipment
    - Herb Drying Racks or Screens: Ensure proper air circulation to prevent mold.
    - Glass Jars with Airtight Lids: For storing dried herbs, protecting them from moisture and light.
    - Labels and Markers: To document the herb's name, date of harvest, and intended use.

- Preparation Tools
    - Mortar and Pestle: For grinding and crushing herbs into powders or pastes.
    - Graters and Peelers: Useful for processing roots and barks like ginger and cinnamon.

Blenders or Food Processors: Modern alternatives for creating purees or powdered forms of herbs.

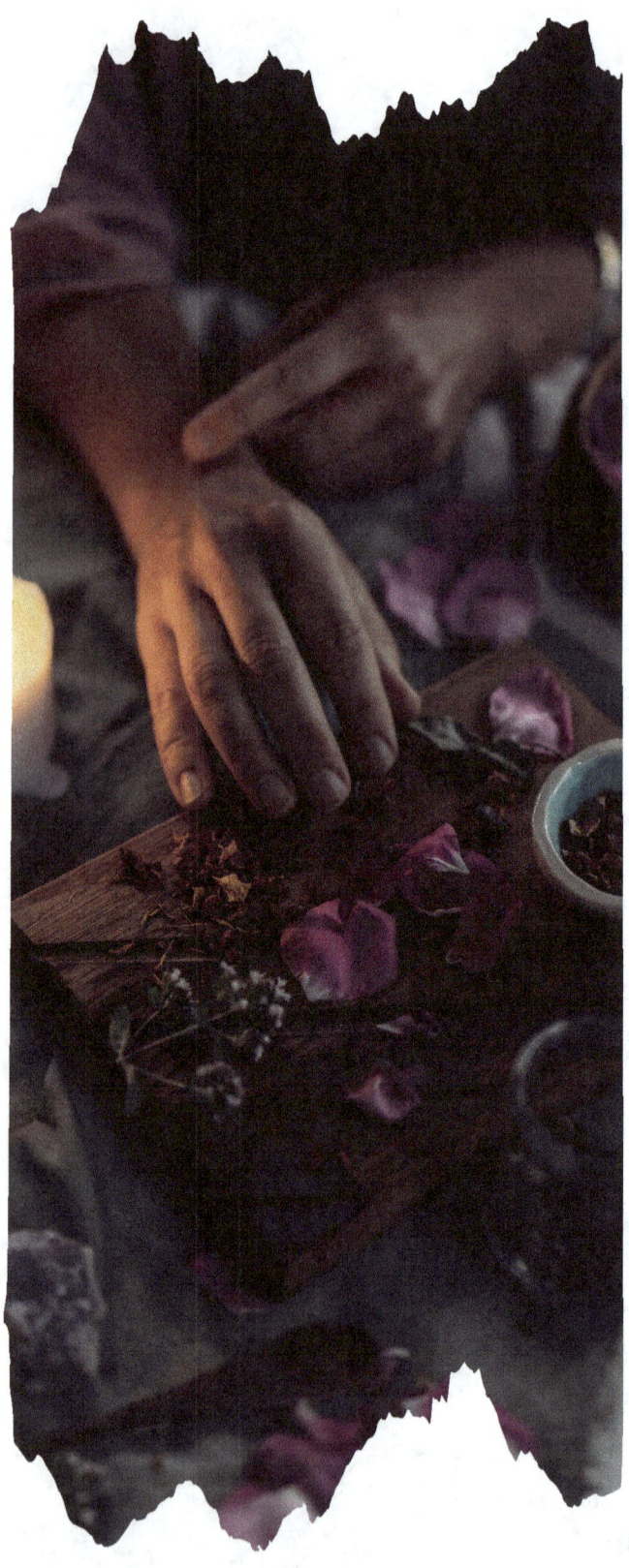

-
- **Double Boiler:** For gently heating herbs to make salves, ointments, or infused oils.
- **Cheesecloth or Fine Mesh Strainer:** To strain herbal infusions, decoctions, or tinctures.
- **Measuring Spoons and Cups:** Ensure accurate dosages when mixing herbal preparations.

1. **Application Tools**
   - **Glass Droppers and Bottles:** For storing tinctures and essential oils.
   - **Compress Cloths or Pads:** For applying herbal compresses.
   - **Reusable Tea Bags or Infusers:** For brewing herbal teas.
2. **Cleaning and Sanitizing Supplies**
   - **Ethanol or Isopropyl Alcohol:** For sterilizing tools and containers.
   - **Boiling Water or Steam:** To ensure equipment remains free of contaminants.

Unique Regional Ingredients and Their Applications

The diversity of herbs used worldwide reflects the unique ecosystems and cultural practices of different regions. Here are some distinctive ingredients and their traditional applications:

1. Africa
    - Baobab Fruit: Rich in vitamin C, used to boost immunity and improve digestion.
    - Moringa Leaves: Known as the "miracle tree," used for energy and anti-inflammatory properties.
    - Kigelia (Sausage Tree): Applied topically for skin conditions and infections.
2. Asia
    - Turmeric (India): A cornerstone of Ayurveda, used for inflammation and joint health.
    - Ginseng (China/Korea): Known for its adaptogenic properties, aiding in stress and energy regulation.
    - Galangal (Southeast Asia): Used for digestive health and as a warming herb in teas.
3. Europe
    - Chamomile (Germany): Popular for relaxation and alleviating digestive discomfort.
    - St. John's Wort (Mediterranean): Known for its use in treating mild depression and nerve pain.
    - Elderberry: Used for its antiviral properties, particularly in fighting colds and flu.
4. North America
    - Echinacea: Widely used for boosting the immune system and preventing infections.
    - Willow Bark: A natural source of salicylic acid, used for pain relief and reducing fever.
    - Black Cohosh: Traditionally used by Native Americans for menopause symptoms and hormonal balance.

5. **South America**
    - **Cat's Claw (Amazon Rainforest):** Known for its anti-inflammatory and immune-boosting effects.
    - **Yerba Mate (Argentina/Paraguay):** A stimulant herb that promotes mental clarity and energy.
    - **Camu Camu:** A superfood packed with vitamin C, supporting immunity and skin health.

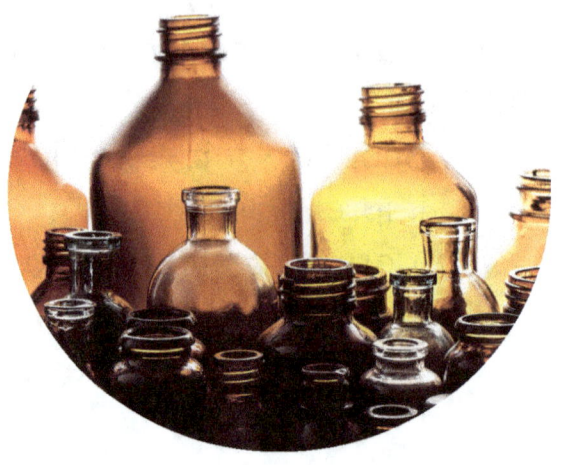

6. **Oceania and Polynesia**
    - **Kava (Pacific Islands):** Used as a ceremonial drink and for reducing anxiety and promoting relaxation.
    - **Tea Tree (Australia):** A potent antimicrobial used in skincare and treating infections.
    - **Non-timber Forest Herbs:** Indigenous plants for balancing mood and improving overall wellness.

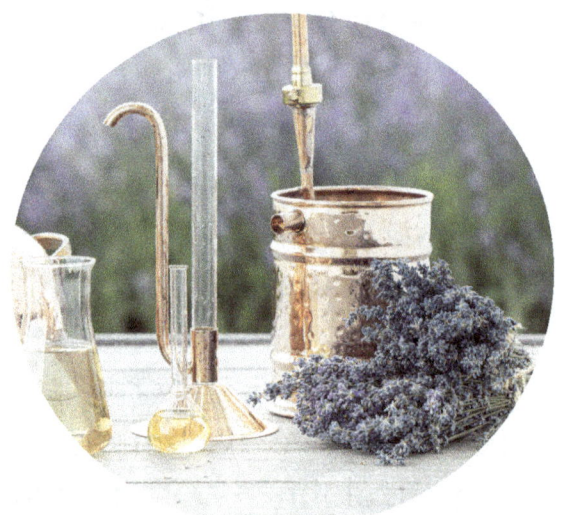

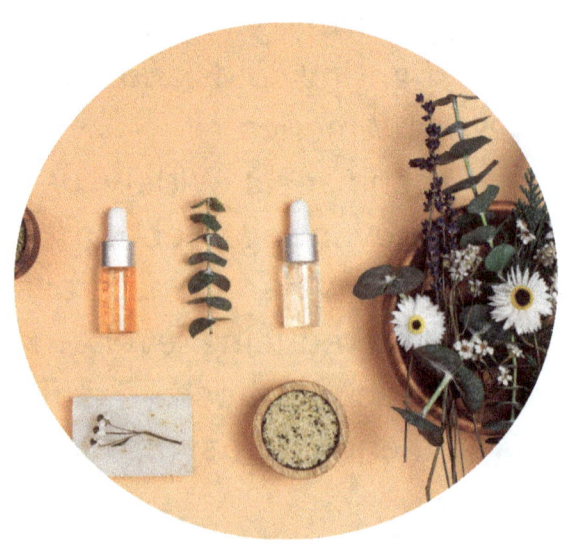

Bringing It Together: Practical Tips
1. Pairing Tools and Ingredients:
2. For instance, a mortar and pestle are ideal for grinding roots like turmeric or galangal, while a fine mesh strainer ensures a smooth tea or infusion from delicate flowers like chamomile or elderberry.
3. Understanding Local Substitutes:
4. If you lack access to regional herbs, research local alternatives that offer similar properties. For example, ginger may substitute galangal in teas or ointments.
5. Combining Wisdom and Modern Techniques:
6. Embrace both traditional methods like slow decoctions for roots and modern approaches such as using food processors for efficiency.
7. Sustainability Practices:
8. Focus on using ethically sourced herbs and reusable tools to minimize waste. Learn from indigenous practices that emphasize harmony with nature.

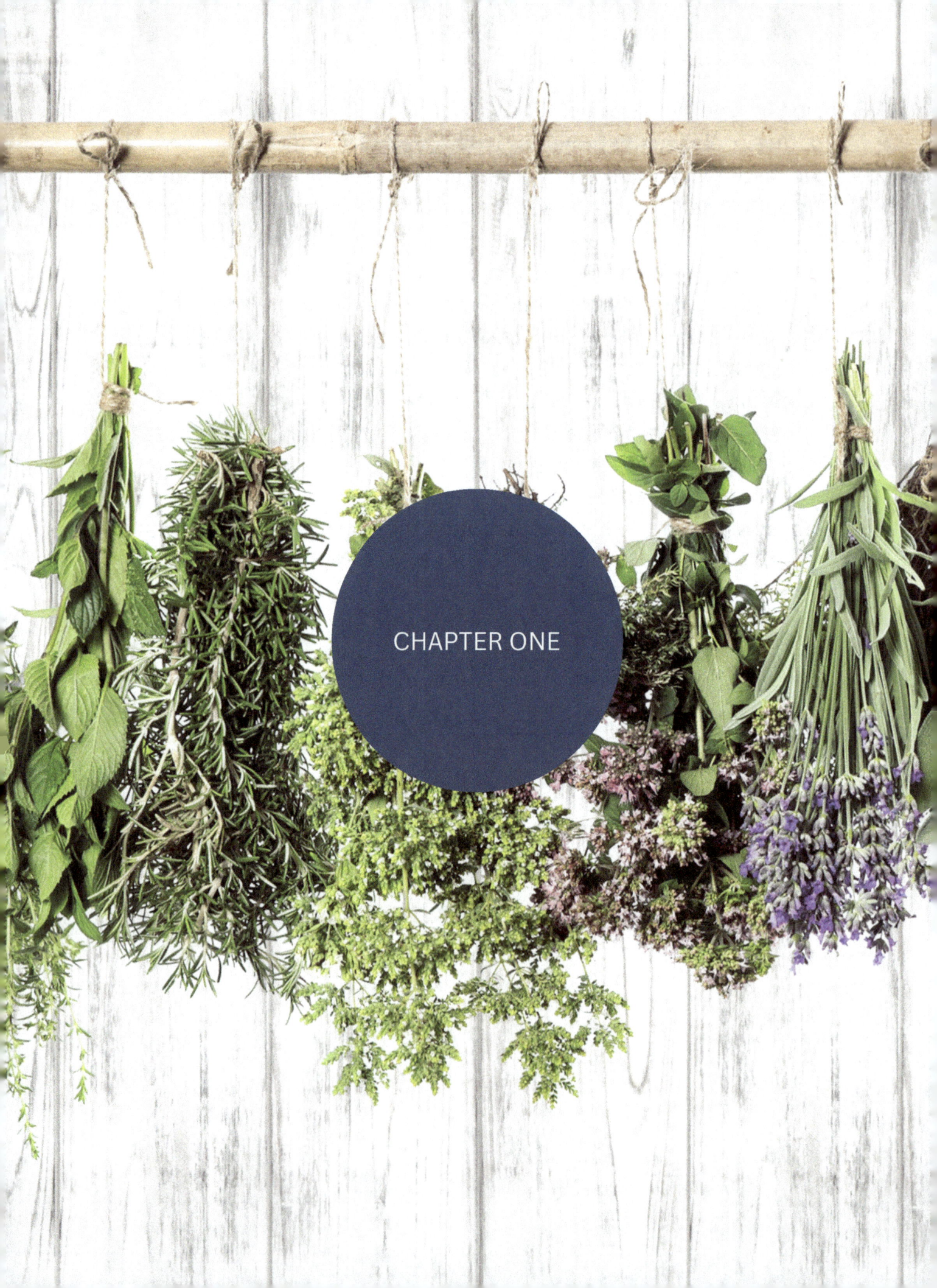

CHAPTER ONE

Understanding Herbal Medicine

Herbal medicine is one of the oldest forms of healthcare, with roots in every culture across the globe. It relies on the therapeutic properties of plants to treat, prevent, and manage various ailments. Modern herbalism bridges traditional knowledge with scientific research, offering a deeper understanding of how plant compounds interact with the human body.

Active Plant Compounds and Their Benefits

Plants produce a vast array of chemical compounds that play critical roles in their survival and in the healing of human ailments. These active compounds, known as phytochemicals, are responsible for the medicinal properties of herbs. Below are some key categories of active plant compounds and their benefits:

1. Alkaloids
   - Description: Nitrogen-containing compounds that have strong physiological effects.
   - Examples and Benefits:
     - Morphine (from opium poppy): Powerful pain reliever.
     - Quinine (from cinchona bark): Treats malaria.
     - Caffeine (from coffee and tea): Stimulates the central nervous system and enhances focus.
2. Flavonoids
   - Description: Antioxidant compounds that protect cells from damage.
   - Examples and Benefits:
     - Quercetin (found in onions and apples): Anti-inflammatory and immune-boosting.

Catechins (in green tea): Promote cardiovascular health and may reduce cancer risk.

3. Terpenes and Terpenoids
    - Description: Aromatic compounds responsible for the scents of many herbs.
    - Examples and Benefits:
        - Menthol (from peppermint): Soothes respiratory issues and relieves pain.
        - Limonene (from citrus fruits): Mood enhancer and digestive aid.
4. Saponins
    - Description: Foam-producing compounds that support immune function.
    - Examples and Benefits:
        - Ginsenosides (from ginseng): Adaptogenic properties that help the body manage stress.
        - Diosgenin (from wild yam): Used as a precursor for steroid hormone synthesis.
5. Phenolic Compounds
    - Description: Include a broad range of antioxidants with protective effects.
    - Examples and Benefits:
        - Tannins (in witch hazel and tea): Astringent properties to treat wounds and inflammation.
        - Curcumin (in turmeric): Anti-inflammatory and supports joint health.
6. Essential Oils
    - Description: Concentrated volatile compounds that provide fragrance and therapeutic effects.
    - Examples and Benefits:
        - Lavender Oil: Promotes relaxation and reduces anxiety.

Tea Tree Oil: Antimicrobial properties for skin care and infection prevention.

7. Glycosides
Description: Compounds that release active substances when metabolized.
1. Examples and Benefits:
2. Salicin (from willow bark): Converts to salicylic acid, a precursor of aspirin, for pain relief.
3. Cardiac Glycosides (from foxglove): Regulates heart rhythm

The Science of Healing Plants
Modern science has validated many traditional uses of herbs by uncovering the mechanisms behind their therapeutic effects. Understanding the science of healing plants bridges the gap between ancient practices and contemporary medicine.
1. **Mechanisms of Action**
    - **Synergistic Effects:** Active compounds often work together to enhance effectiveness. For example, the combination of flavonoids and tannins in green tea improves its antioxidant properties.
    - **Targeted Action:** Certain compounds bind to specific receptors in the body. For instance, alkaloids like morphine bind to opioid receptors to relieve pain.
2. **Bioavailability and Absorption**
    - Herbs differ in how their compounds are absorbed by the body. For example:
        - *Curcumin* (from turmeric) has low bioavailability but can be enhanced with black pepper (piperine).
        - *Fat-soluble compounds* (like those in chamomile) are better absorbed with dietary fats.
3. **Dosage and Safety**
    - Effective herbal remedies depend on proper dosages. For instance, while ginseng is beneficial in moderate amounts, excessive use can lead to overstimulation.
    - Understanding potential interactions with medications is critical. For example, St. John's Wort can reduce the efficacy of certain

drugs, such as oral contraceptives.
4. **Research and Validation**
   - The therapeutic effects of herbs are often confirmed through clinical studies. Examples include:
     - *Echinacea:* Found to shorten the duration of colds.
     - *Garlic:* Shown to reduce blood pressure and cholesterol levels.
   - *Ethnobotanical Studies:* Document how indigenous communities use plants, guiding pharmaceutical research.
5. **The Role of Microbiota**
   - Recent studies reveal that gut bacteria can metabolize herbal compounds, enhancing or modifying their effects. For instance, the conversion of flavonoids into bioactive forms depends on a healthy gut microbiome.

Integrating Herbal Medicine into Modern Practices
1. **Standardized Extracts:**
   - Advances in extraction techniques ensure consistent potency, making herbal medicine more reliable.
   - For example, standardized ginkgo biloba extracts are used for cognitive enhancement.
2. **Combination Therapies:**
   - Herbs are increasingly being combined with conventional treatments. For instance, using ginger to alleviate nausea caused by chemotherapy.
3. **Personalized Herbalism:**
   - Advances in genetic testing and microbiome analysis are paving the way for personalized herbal therapies tailored to an individual's needs.
4. **Preservation of Traditional Knowledge:**
   - Collaborations between scientists and indigenous communities ensure the sustainable use of plant resources while honoring cultural heritage.

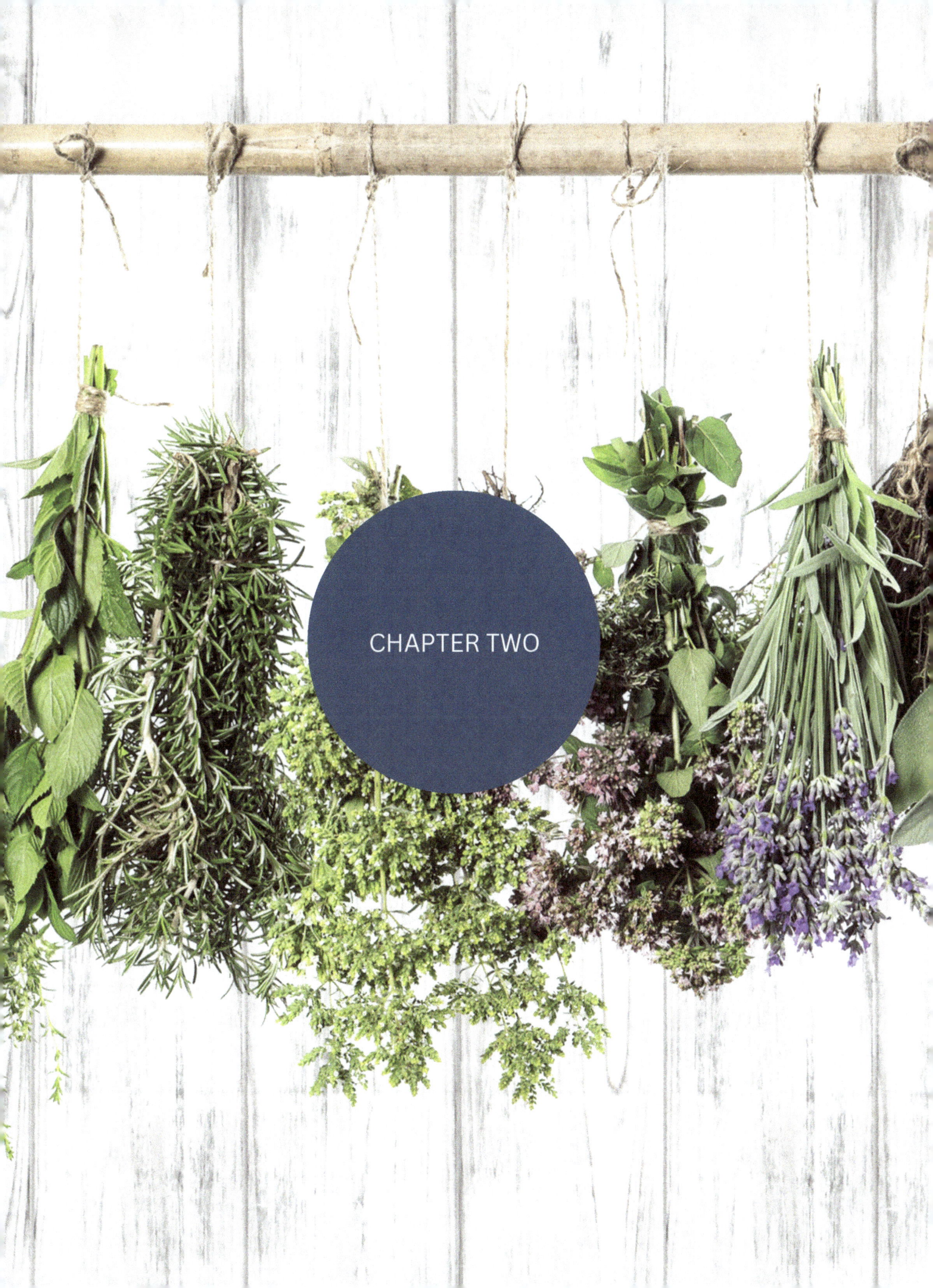

CHAPTER TWO

African Herbal Traditions

Africa's rich biodiversity has fostered a deep and enduring tradition of herbal medicine. Across the continent, indigenous knowledge of medicinal plants has been passed down through generations, forming the foundation of health and healing practices in both rural and urban communities. African herbal medicine is not just about physical healing—it is intertwined with cultural, spiritual, and social aspects of life, reflecting the holistic nature of traditional practices.

Key Herbs and Their Uses
1. Moringa (Nutrient Boost)
    - Scientific Name: Moringa oleifera
    - Description: Often referred to as the "miracle tree," moringa is native to parts of West Africa and widely cultivated across the continent. Its leaves, seeds, and pods are packed with essential nutrients.
    - Medicinal Uses:
        - High in vitamins A, C, and E, as well as minerals like iron and calcium, moringa is a natural multivitamin.
        - Used to combat malnutrition, especially in children and nursing mothers.
        - Has antioxidant properties that reduce oxidative stress and inflammation.
        - Supports liver function and detoxification.
        - Research suggests it may help regulate blood sugar levels, making it beneficial for diabetics.
    - Preparation:
        - The dried leaves are ground into powder and added to food or drinks.
        - Fresh leaves are used in soups and stews.
        - Moringa oil, extracted from seeds, is used for skincare and wound healing.

2. Baobab (Immunity and Digestive Health)
    - Scientific Name: Adansonia digitata
    - Description: Known as the "tree of life," the baobab is revered for its fruit, which has a high concentration of vitamin C, fiber, and antioxidants.
    - Medicinal Uses:
        - Strengthens the immune system, thanks to its high vitamin C content.
        - The fiber in baobab fruit promotes digestive health by supporting gut microbiota.
        - Its anti-inflammatory properties are used to manage asthma and allergies.
        - Helps in hydration and electrolyte balance, especially in hot climates.
    - Preparation:
        - The dried fruit pulp is made into a powder and mixed with water to create a refreshing drink.
        - Used in porridges and smoothies.
        - The bark and leaves are boiled into teas for respiratory ailments.
2. Devil's Claw (Joint Pain Relief)
    - Scientific Name: Harpagophytum procumbens
    - Description: Native to Southern Africa, this herb is renowned for its hooked fruit and powerful anti-inflammatory properties.
    - Medicinal Uses:
        - Effective in reducing joint pain and stiffness associated with arthritis and rheumatism.
        - Alleviates lower back pain and muscle soreness.
        - Acts as a digestive stimulant and appetite enhancer.
        - Research supports its use in managing osteoarthritis symptoms.
    - Preparation:

- The dried root is brewed into teas or made into tinctures.
- Extracts are incorporated into capsules or topical creams for pain relief.
- **Cultural Use:**
  - Traditionally used by the San and Khoikhoi peoples for wound healing and fever reduction.

4. **Hibiscus (Blood Pressure Regulation)**
   - **Scientific Name:** *Hibiscus sabdariffa*
   - **Description:** Widely grown in West Africa, hibiscus flowers are vibrant and packed with flavonoids and anthocyanins.
   - **Medicinal Uses:**
     - Lowers blood pressure and improves cardiovascular health.
     - A natural diuretic, helping to reduce water retention.
     - Has antimicrobial properties that support oral health.
     - Contains antioxidants that combat free radicals and prevent chronic diseases.
   - **Preparation:**
     - The dried petals are steeped to make a tangy, ruby-red tea, often sweetened with honey.
     - Combined with spices like ginger and cloves for a warming infusion.
   - **Cultural Use:**
     - Known as *Zobo* in Nigeria, it is a popular drink served at celebrations.

5. **Neem (Antiviral and Antibacterial Properties)**
   - **Scientific Name:** *Azadirachta indica*
   - **Description:** Originating from West Africa and India, neem is a versatile herb used for centuries in African and Asian medicine.
   - **Medicinal Uses:**
     - Antiviral and antibacterial properties make it effective against infections and skin conditions.
     - Neem oil is used to treat eczema, psoriasis, and acne.

Supports oral hygiene by reducing plaque and preventing gum disease.

- Purifies the blood and boosts liver health.
- Neem tea is used to manage fever and respiratory infections.
- **Preparation:**
    - The leaves are boiled to make teas or ground into pastes for topical application.
    - Neem oil, extracted from seeds, is used in massage therapy and skincare.
- **Cultural Use:**
    - In African traditional medicine, neem leaves are often placed around homes to ward off mosquitoes and other pests.

Indigenous Herbal Practices
1. **Cultural Healing Systems**
    - Across Africa, herbal medicine is often practiced within the framework of traditional healing systems, such as Yoruba *Ifa* medicine in Nigeria, Zulu healing traditions in South Africa, and Berber herbalism in North Africa.
    - Healers, known as herbalists or *sangomas*, play a dual role as medical practitioners and spiritual guides.
    - Herbs are often combined with spiritual rituals, prayers, and ancestral invocations to treat both physical and metaphysical ailments.
2. **Herbal Formulations**
    - Many African herbal remedies are multi-herb preparations, where different plants are combined for synergistic effects.
        - Example: A mixture of *kinkeliba* (Combretum micranthum) and baobab for fever and hydration.

Herbal baths and steams are used for skin disorders and respiratory issues.

- **Preservation of Knowledge**
    - Knowledge of herbal medicine is passed down orally, often through apprenticeship.
    - Increasingly, there are efforts to document this knowledge to preserve it for future generations and integrate it into global healthcare systems.
- **Sustainability and Conservation**
    - With the growing demand for medicinal plants, sustainability practices are essential to prevent overharvesting.
    - Community-based cultivation and protection of sacred groves help preserve biodiversity.

African herbal traditions represent a treasure trove of knowledge, with countless herbs offering therapeutic benefits that modern science continues to validate. Incorporating these practices into contemporary herbal medicine ensures that this wisdom endures, benefiting people worldwide.

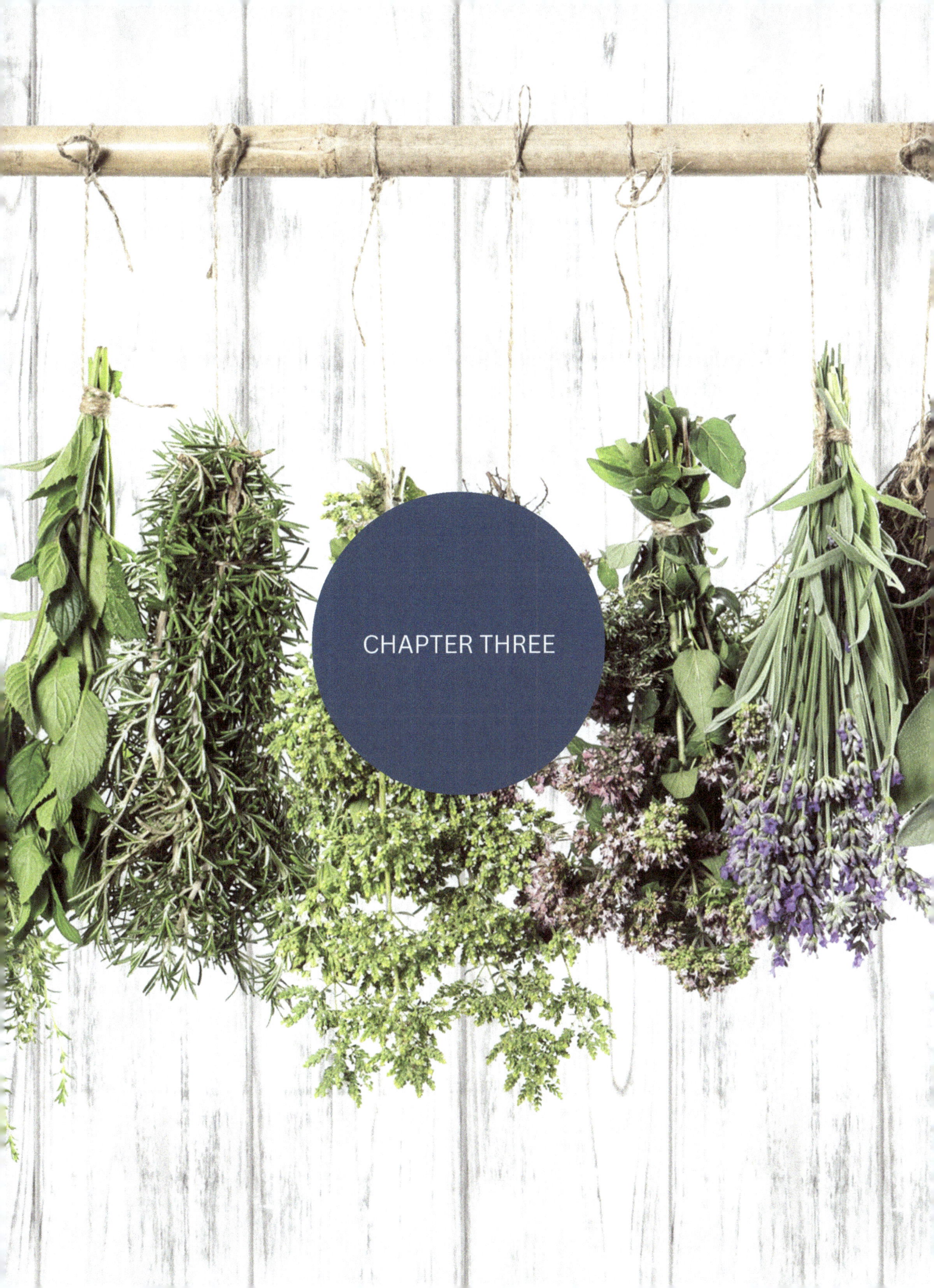

CHAPTER THREE

Asian Herbal Traditions

Asia is home to some of the most ancient and sophisticated systems of herbal medicine, including Traditional Chinese Medicine (TCM), Ayurveda, and the rich herbal traditions of Southeast Asia. These systems are deeply rooted in a holistic understanding of health, where the mind, body, and spirit are interconnected. Each tradition emphasizes balance, harmony, and the use of herbs to support the body's natural healing processes.

Chinese, Indian (Ayurvedic), and Southeast Asian Contributions

- **Traditional Chinese Medicine (TCM):** Developed over 2,000 years, TCM emphasizes the balance of *yin* and *yang* and the smooth flow of *qi* (vital energy) through the body.
- Herbs are used in combination, often in formulas tailored to individual constitutions and conditions.
- Key TCM remedies include herbs like ginseng, licorice root, and astragalus, often used alongside acupuncture and dietary therapy.
- **Ayurveda:** Originating in India over 3,000 years ago, Ayurveda focuses on balancing the three *doshas* (Vata, Pitta, Kapha) that govern the body and mind.
- Ayurvedic herbal medicine uses plants such as turmeric, holy basil, and ashwagandha to address imbalances and promote overall health.
- Preparation methods include teas, powders, and oil infusions, often combined with yoga and meditation.

1. Southeast Asian Herbal Medicine
   - This region's herbal traditions are a fusion of influences from Chinese, Indian, and indigenous practices.
   - Herbs like ginger, lemongrass, and gotu kola are widely used for their culinary and medicinal properties.
   - Herbal steams and baths are a hallmark of healing traditions in countries like Thailand and Indonesia.

Key Herbs and Their Uses
1. Ginseng (Vitality and Energy)
   - Scientific Name: Panax ginseng (Asian Ginseng)
   - Description: A revered herb in TCM, ginseng is known as the "root of immortality." Its adaptogenic properties make it one of the most sought-after herbs for boosting energy and resilience.
   - Medicinal Uses:
     - Enhances physical and mental stamina.
     - Reduces stress and promotes overall vitality.
     - Improves cognitive function and memory.
     - Strengthens the immune system and supports recovery from illness.
   - Preparation:
     - Sliced root is brewed into teas.
     - Powdered ginseng is added to soups or taken in capsules.
     - Often combined with other herbs in TCM formulas for tailored benefits.
2. Turmeric (Anti-Inflammatory)
   - Scientific Name: Curcuma longa
   - Description: A staple in Ayurvedic and Southeast Asian medicine, turmeric is valued for its vibrant yellow pigment and potent health benefits.

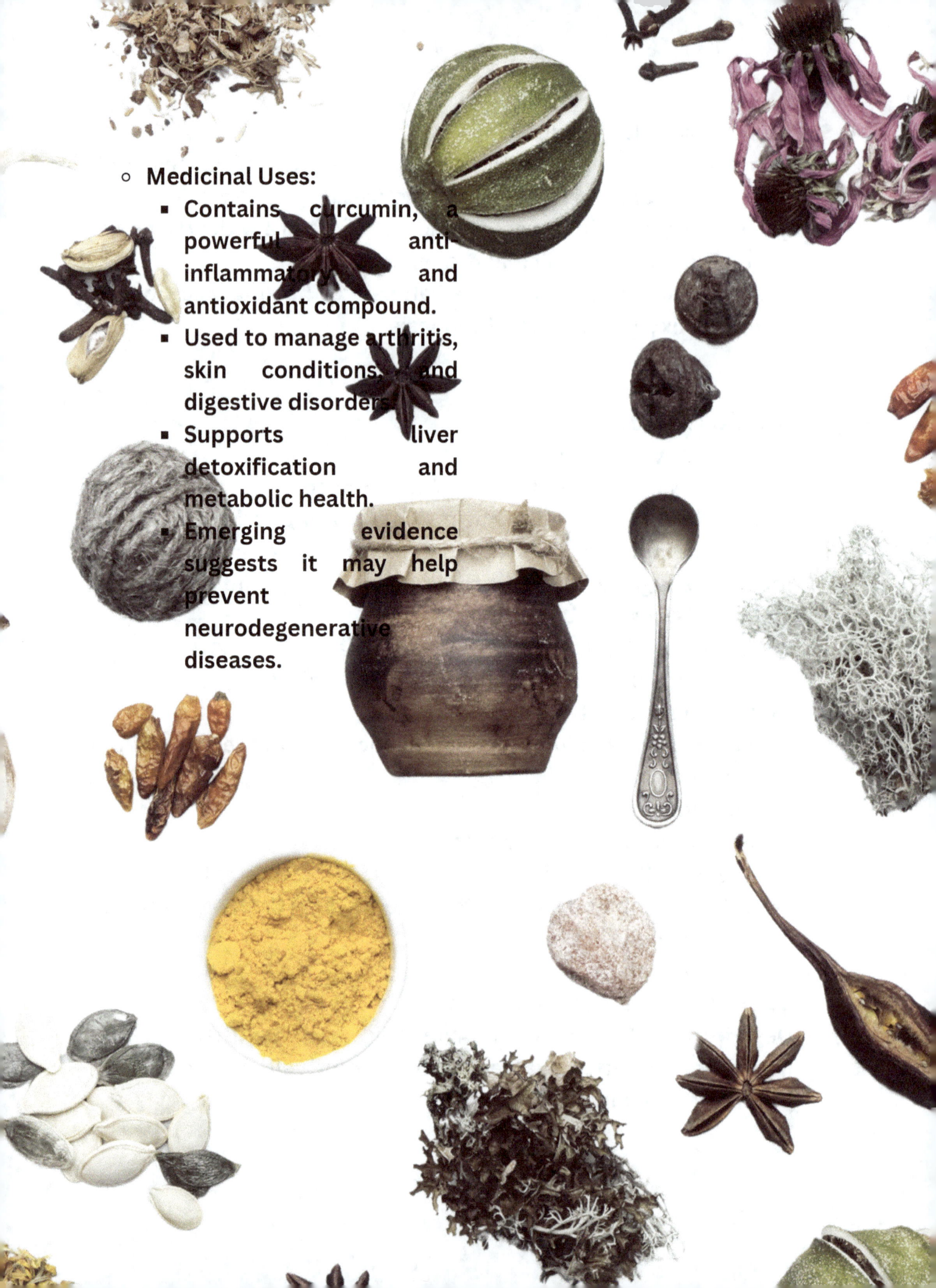

- Medicinal Uses:
  - Contains curcumin, a powerful anti-inflammatory and antioxidant compound.
  - Used to manage arthritis, skin conditions, and digestive disorders.
  - Supports liver detoxification and metabolic health.
  - Emerging evidence suggests it may help prevent neurodegenerative diseases.

- **Preparation:**
  - Fresh or dried rhizomes are ground into powder and used in cooking or teas.
  - Golden milk (turmeric latte) is a popular Ayurvedic preparation.
  - Combined with black pepper to enhance bioavailability.

1. **Gotu Kola (Cognitive Health)**
   - **Scientific Name:** *Centella asiatica*
   - **Description:** Widely used in Southeast Asia and Ayurveda, gotu kola is known as a "brain tonic" for its ability to enhance mental clarity and reduce anxiety.
   - **Medicinal Uses:**
     - Improves memory, concentration, and cognitive function.
     - Promotes wound healing and reduces scarring.
     - Alleviates symptoms of anxiety and stress.
     - Strengthens blood vessels and improves circulation, especially in varicose veins.

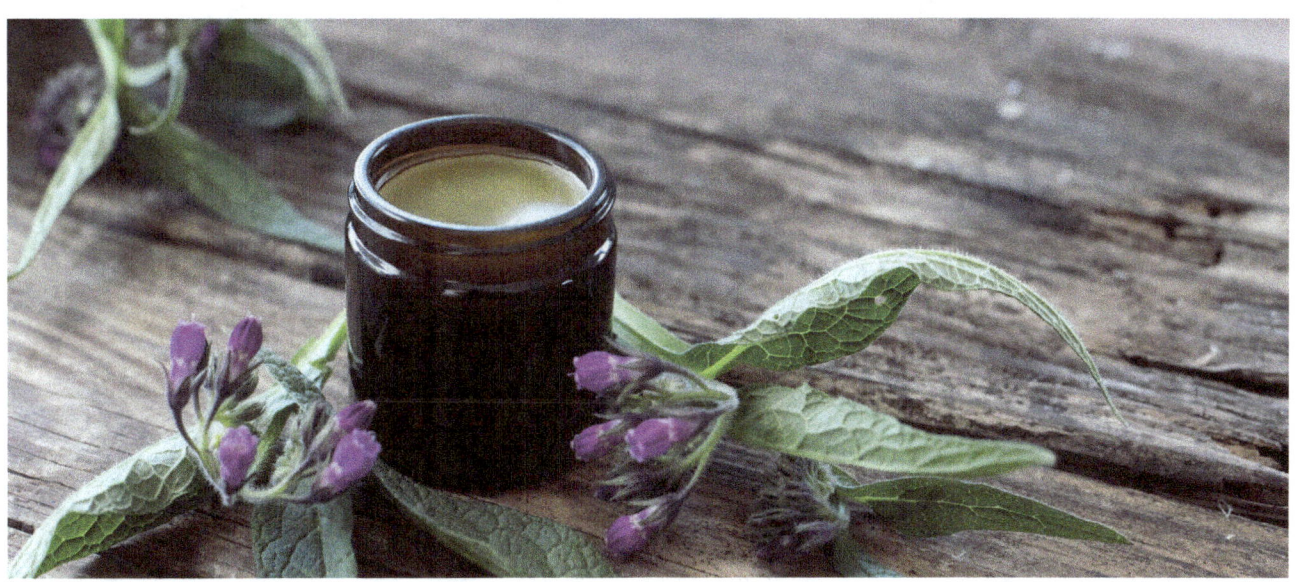

- **Preparation:**
  - Leaves are eaten fresh, brewed into teas, or made into extracts.
  - Often used in herbal salves for topical applications.
- **Licorice Root (Digestive Aid)**
  - **Scientific Name:** *Glycyrrhiza glabra*
  - **Description:** A versatile herb in TCM and Ayurveda, licorice root is prized for its sweet taste and soothing properties.
  - **Medicinal Uses:**
    - Soothes digestive discomfort and reduces acid reflux.
    - Acts as an expectorant for coughs and sore throats.
    - Supports adrenal health and reduces fatigue.
    - Anti-inflammatory properties make it useful in skin conditions like eczema.
  - **Preparation:**
    - Dried root is boiled into decoctions or added to herbal teas.
    - Extracts are used in syrups and lozenges.
    - Often included in multi-herb formulations to enhance their effectiveness.

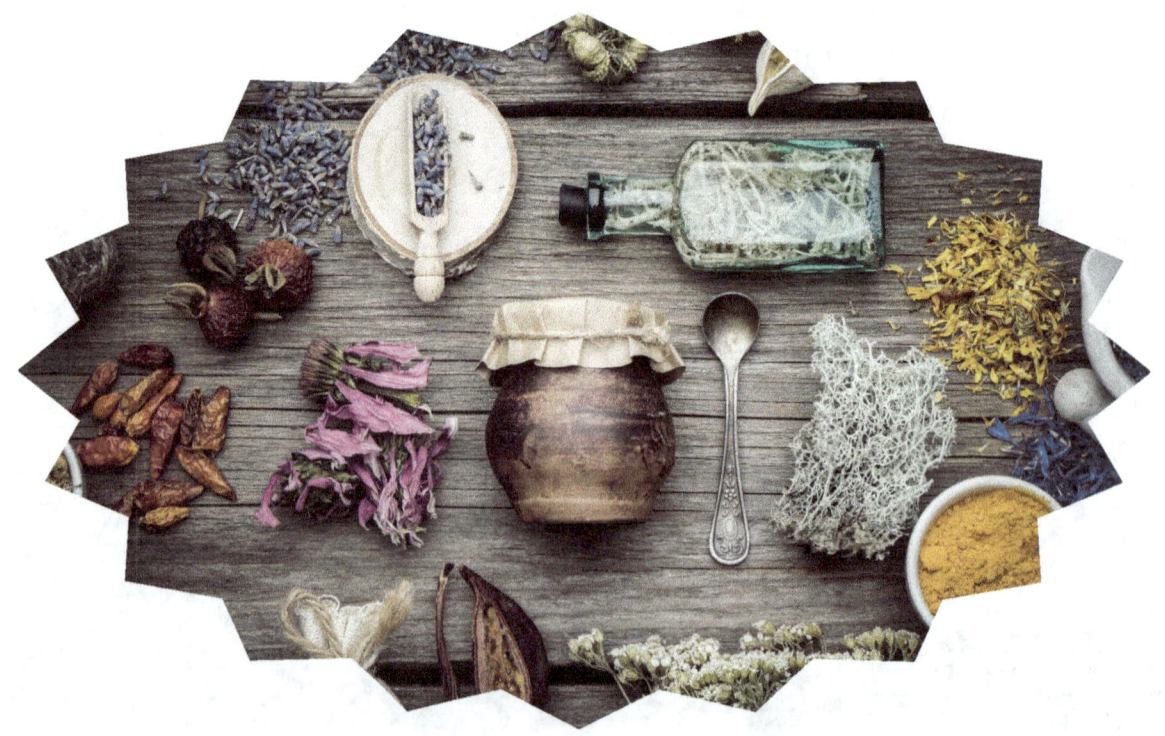

1. **Holy Basil (Tulsi) (Stress Relief)**
   - **Scientific Name:** *Ocimum sanctum*
   - **Description:** Considered sacred in Ayurveda, tulsi is an adaptogen that helps the body adapt to stress and maintain balance.
   - **Medicinal Uses:**
     - Reduces cortisol levels, alleviating stress and anxiety.
     - Supports respiratory health and immune function.
     - Antimicrobial properties help prevent infections.
     - Improves cardiovascular health by reducing cholesterol and blood pressure.
   - **Preparation:**
     - Fresh leaves are brewed into teas or eaten raw.
     - Tulsi oil is used for aromatherapy and topical applications.
     - Dried leaves are powdered and encapsulated for supplementation.

These key herbs exemplify the diversity and potency of Asian herbal medicine. Through centuries of refinement, the practices from this region have significantly influenced modern herbal therapies, providing remedies that address not just physical ailments but also emotional and spiritual well-being.

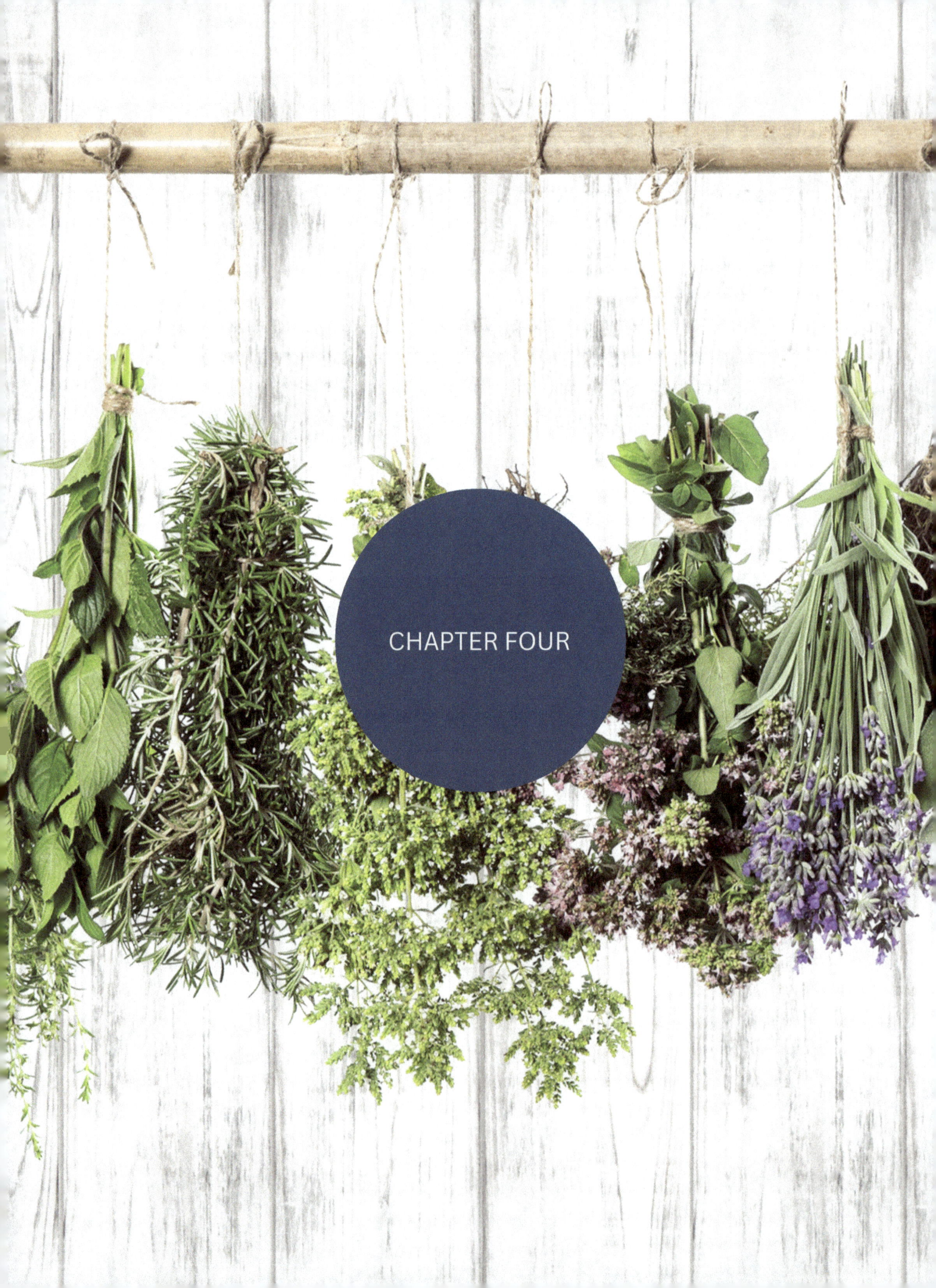

CHAPTER FOUR

European Herbal Traditions

Europe boasts a rich history of herbal medicine, tracing its roots from the ancient civilizations of Greece and Rome to the flourishing herbal traditions of the medieval period and modern herbalism. European practices emphasize both scientific inquiry and traditional wisdom, blending the healing power of nature with contemporary research. This chapter explores the evolution of herbal traditions in Europe and highlights key herbs that have stood the test of time.

From Ancient Rome to Modern Herbalism
1. Ancient Rome and Greece
    - Early European herbalism was shaped significantly by the works of Greek physicians like Hippocrates and Dioscorides.
    - The Roman Empire adopted Greek medicinal practices, documenting herbal remedies in texts like De Materia Medica by Dioscorides.
    - Popular herbs included thyme, rosemary, and chamomile, used for their medicinal and culinary properties.
2. Medieval Herbalism
    - The medieval period saw the rise of herbal gardens maintained by monasteries. Monks and nuns cultivated medicinal plants and recorded their uses in herbals (manuscripts detailing the properties of plants).
    - Hildegard of Bingen, a Benedictine abbess, was a prominent herbalist who combined spiritual and medical knowledge in her writings.
3. The Renaissance and Beyond
    - The Renaissance era brought renewed interest in herbal medicine, with the invention of the printing press facilitating the widespread dissemination of herbal knowledge.
    - Nicholas Culpeper, an English herbalist, wrote The Complete Herbal, which emphasized using local plants for healing.

4. Modern European Herbalism
    - Today, European herbal medicine integrates traditional practices with evidence-based approaches. Herbal remedies are used alongside modern medicine, particularly in countries like Germany and the UK.
    - The European Union regulates herbal medicines to ensure safety and efficacy, with a focus on standardizing herbal extracts.

Key Herbs and Their Uses
  1. Lavender (Relaxation and Skin Care)
     - Scientific Name: Lavandula angustifolia
     - Description: Lavender has been cherished since Roman times for its calming aroma and healing properties.
     - Medicinal Uses:
       - Promotes relaxation and reduces anxiety.
       - Improves sleep quality and alleviates insomnia.
       - Treats minor burns, cuts, and skin irritations.
       - Helps relieve headaches and migraines when applied topically.
     - Preparation:
       - Dried flowers are infused into teas or used in sachets for aromatherapy.
       - Lavender oil is applied topically or added to baths for relaxation.
  2. Chamomile (Sleep Aid and Digestive Soother)
     - Scientific Name: Matricaria chamomilla
     - Description: A staple in European herbalism, chamomile is known for its gentle and soothing properties.

Medicinal Uses:
- Alleviates insomnia and promotes restful sleep.
- Reduces digestive discomfort, including bloating and cramps.
- Soothes skin irritations and eczema.
- Acts as an anti-inflammatory for minor aches and pains.
  - Preparation:
    - Flowers are steeped in hot water to make herbal teas.
    - Chamomile oil is used in skincare and aromatherapy.

3. Elderberry (Immune Support)
   - Scientific Name: Sambucus nigra
   - Description: Elderberry has long been valued in European folk medicine for its immune-boosting properties.
   - Medicinal Uses:
     - Helps reduce the severity and duration of colds and flu.
     - Provides antioxidant support to combat free radicals.
     - Supports respiratory health and relieves sinus congestion.
     - Promotes healthy skin through its anti-inflammatory effects.
   - Preparation:
     - Berries are made into syrups, teas, and tinctures.
     - Flowers are used in infusions or to flavor foods and beverages.

4. St. John's Wort (Mood Enhancement)
   - Scientific Name: Hypericum perforatum
   - Description: This herb has been used for centuries to support mental health and emotional well-being.
   - Medicinal Uses:
     - Acts as a natural antidepressant by boosting serotonin levels.
     - Eases mild to moderate depression and anxiety.
     - Helps with nerve pain and inflammation.
     - Assists in wound healing when applied topically.

- Preparation:
  - Dried flowers are steeped into teas or infused into oils.
  - Extracts are standardized into capsules or tinctures for mental health benefits.

5. Thyme (Antiseptic and Respiratory Health)
   - Scientific Name: Thymus vulgaris
   - Description: Known since Roman times, thyme is a potent herb with antiseptic and expectorant properties.
   - Medicinal Uses:
     - Treats respiratory conditions like coughs, bronchitis, and sore throats.
     - Acts as a natural antiseptic for cleaning wounds.
     - Aids in digestion and alleviates bloating.
     - Supports immune health through its antimicrobial properties.
   - Preparation:
     - Fresh or dried thyme is brewed into teas or added to culinary dishes.
     - Essential oil is used in steam inhalations for respiratory relief.
     - Extracts are incorporated into syrups and lozenges for cough relief.

European herbal traditions offer a wealth of knowledge and remedies that continue to benefit modern health practices. By combining centuries-old wisdom with scientific validation, these traditions provide a holistic approach to healing that remains relevant and effective today.

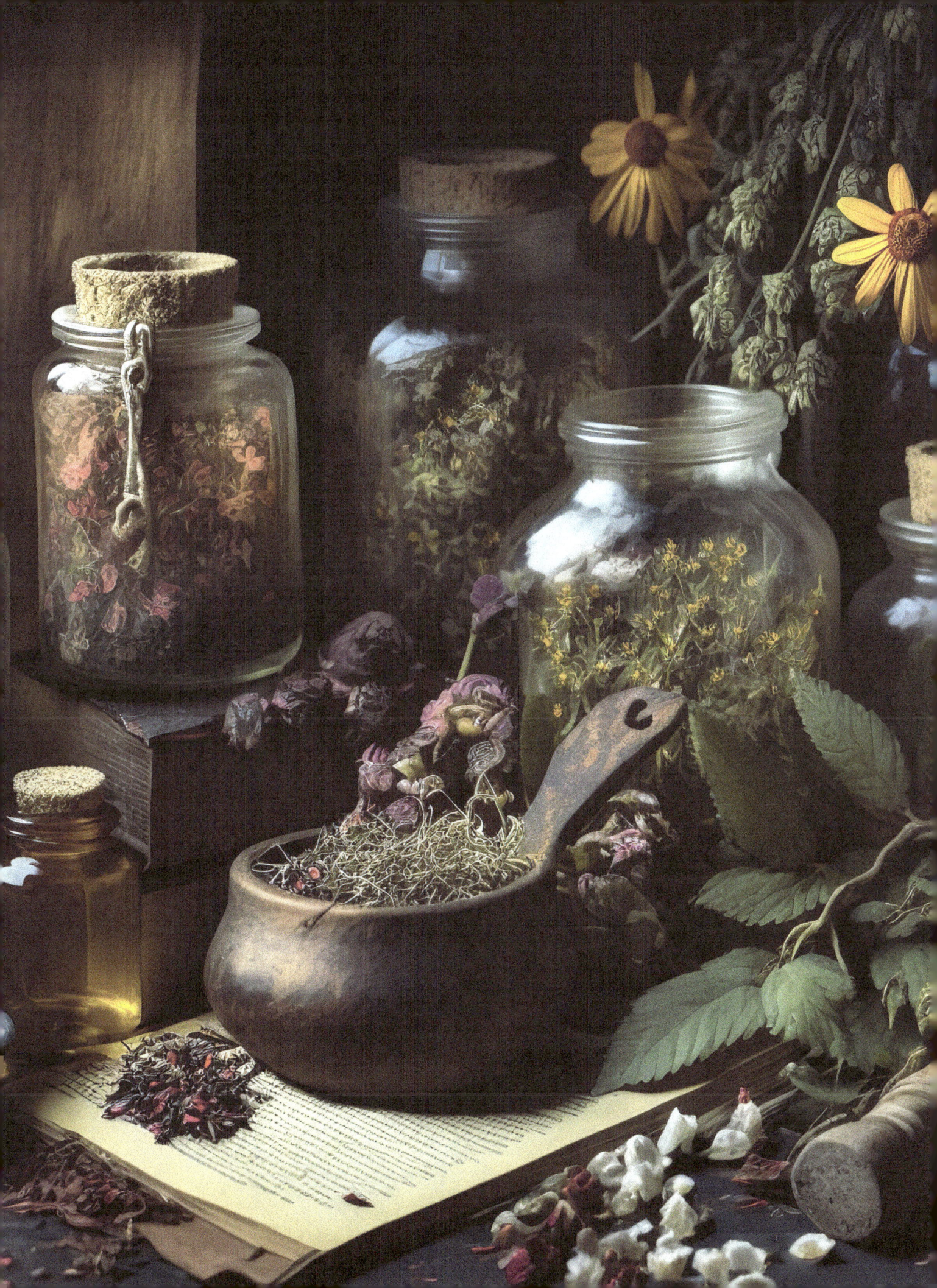

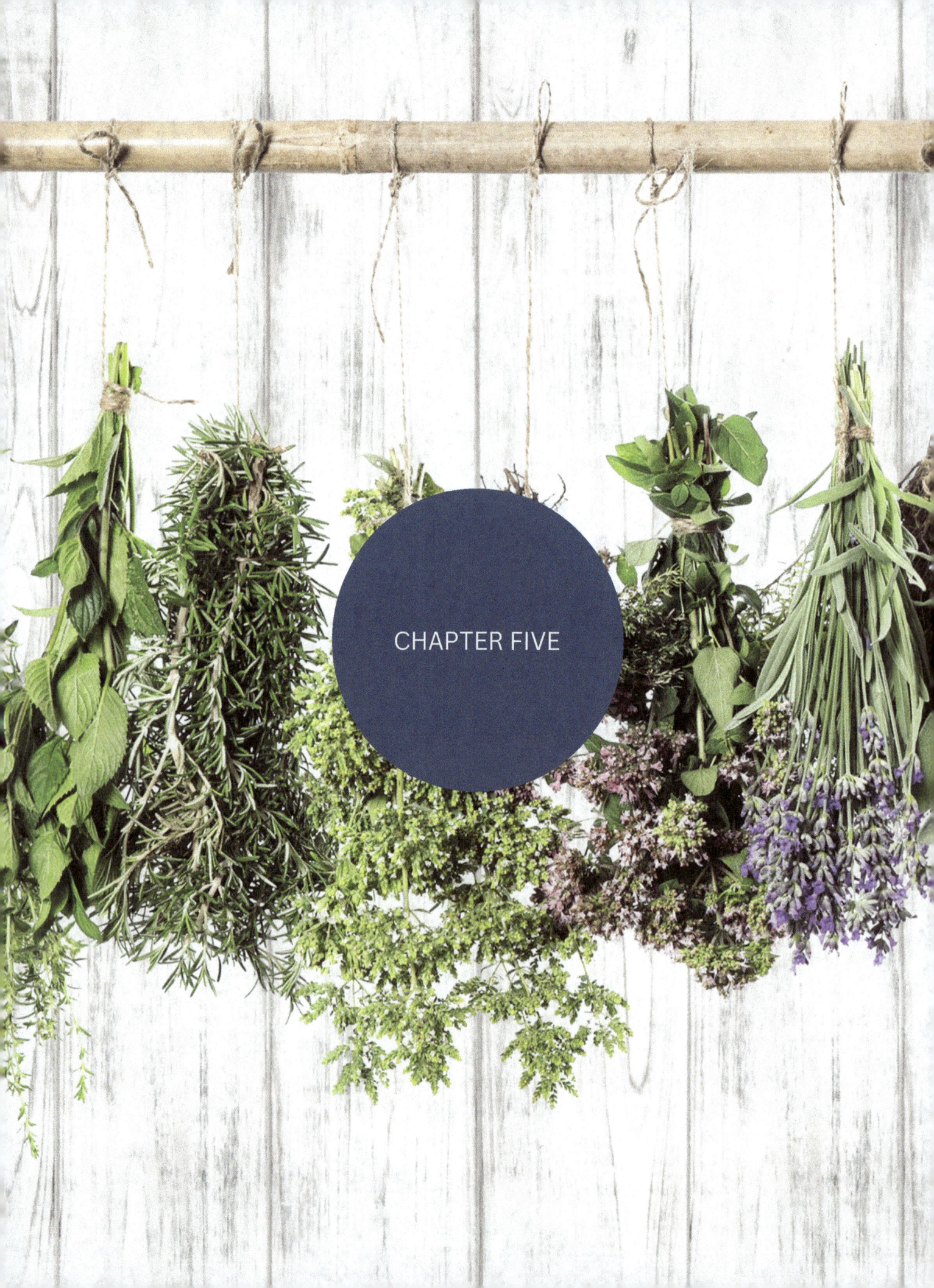

CHAPTER FIVE

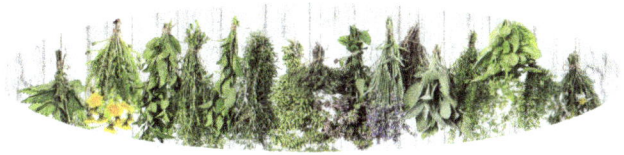 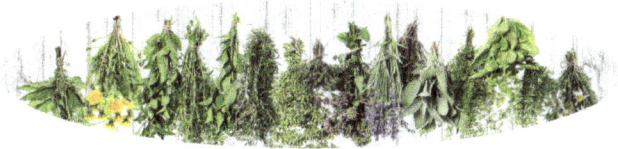

Native American Herbal Traditions

Native American cultures have long revered plants for their sacred and healing properties, using them not only for physical ailments but also as part of spiritual and ceremonial practices. These traditions, passed down orally through generations, represent a deep connection with the land and an understanding of its natural resources. This chapter explores the rich herbal heritage of Native American communities, highlighting sacred plants, their uses, and their enduring relevance.

Sacred Plants of Indigenous Cultures

For Native Americans, plants were more than just remedies—they were gifts from nature, deeply intertwined with spiritual beliefs and rituals. Sacred plants were used to cleanse spaces, connect with the divine, and promote holistic well-being.

1. **Rituals and Ceremonial Use**
   - Plants like sage, cedar, and sweetgrass were burned as part of smudging ceremonies to purify the body, mind, and spirit.
   - Tobacco, considered sacred, was offered during prayers or used in peace pipes to symbolize respect and communication with the Creator.
2. **Healing Philosophy**
   - Native American healing combines physical, emotional, and spiritual health, viewing these aspects as interconnected.
   - Remedies often included chants, prayers, and the use of herbal medicines, reflecting a holistic approach to wellness.

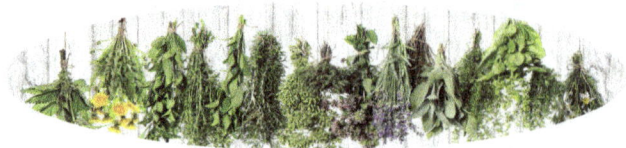
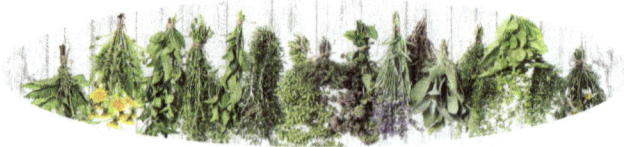

3. Sustainability and Respect for Nature
    - Harvesting was done with gratitude, taking only what was needed and ensuring the plant population remained sustainable.
    - Rituals often included offerings, such as cornmeal, to honor the spirits of the plants.

Key Herbs and Their Uses
  1. Echinacea (Immune Booster)
     - Scientific Name: Echinacea purpurea
     - Description: Also known as coneflower, echinacea was a staple in Native American medicine for its immune-strengthening properties.
     - Medicinal Uses:
       - Enhances immune response to fight infections and colds.
       - Reduces inflammation and speeds up wound healing.
       - Alleviates symptoms of respiratory illnesses.
     - Preparation:
       - Roots and flowers are brewed into teas or tinctures.
       - Poultices made from crushed roots are applied to wounds or insect bites.
  2. Sage (Cleansing and Respiratory Aid)
     - Scientific Name: Salvia officinalis or Artemisia ludoviciana (white sage)
     - Description: Sage is a sacred plant used in smudging rituals to cleanse spaces and energy fields.

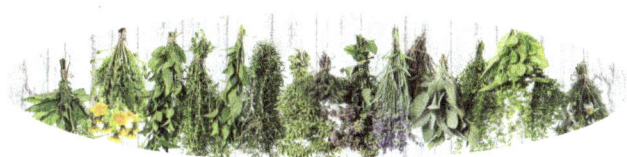
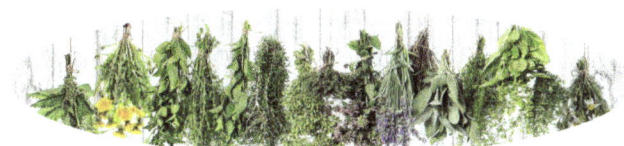

- **Medicinal Uses:**
    - Clears respiratory congestion and supports lung health.
    - Soothes sore throats and reduces inflammation.
    - Acts as an antimicrobial agent for wound care.
- **Preparation:**
    - Leaves are burned for smudging or steeped into teas for respiratory benefits.
    - Infused oils are applied topically for minor skin conditions.

3. **Black Cohosh (Women's Health)**
    - **Scientific Name:** *Actaea racemosa*
    - **Description:** Native Americans used black cohosh for its effects on reproductive health and hormonal balance.
    - **Medicinal Uses:**
        - Alleviates symptoms of menopause, such as hot flashes and mood swings.
        - Relieves menstrual cramps and supports uterine health.
        - Acts as an anti-inflammatory for arthritis and muscle pain.
    - **Preparation:**
        - Roots are dried and brewed into teas or tinctures.
        - Standardized extracts are used for hormonal support.

4. **Willow Bark (Pain Relief)**
    - **Scientific Name:** *Salix alba*
    - **Description:** Known as "nature's aspirin," willow bark contains salicin, a compound later synthesized into modern aspirin.

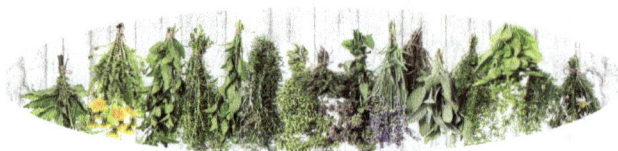
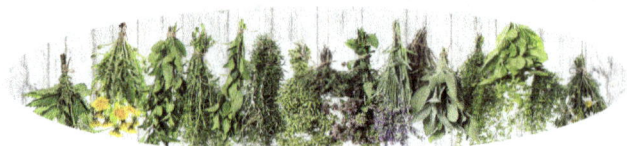

- **Medicinal Uses:**
    - Relieves headaches, muscle pain, and arthritis.
    - Reduces fever and inflammation.
    - Supports cardiovascular health by thinning the blood.
- **Preparation:**
    - Bark is stripped and boiled to create decoctions or teas.
    - Crushed bark is applied as a poultice for localized pain.

5. **Yarrow (Wound Healing)**
    - **Scientific Name:** *Achillea millefolium*
    - **Description:** Yarrow was widely used for its ability to stop bleeding and promote wound healing.
    - **Medicinal Uses:**
        - Stops bleeding and prevents infections in wounds.
        - Eases digestive discomfort and menstrual cramps.
        - Acts as an anti-inflammatory and fever reducer.
    - **Preparation:**
        - Fresh leaves are crushed and applied directly to wounds.
        - Dried flowers and leaves are used to make teas or infusions for internal use.

Native American herbal traditions reflect a profound respect for the natural world and its healing capabilities. These practices continue to inspire modern herbal medicine, offering insights into sustainable living, holistic health, and the spiritual dimensions of healing.

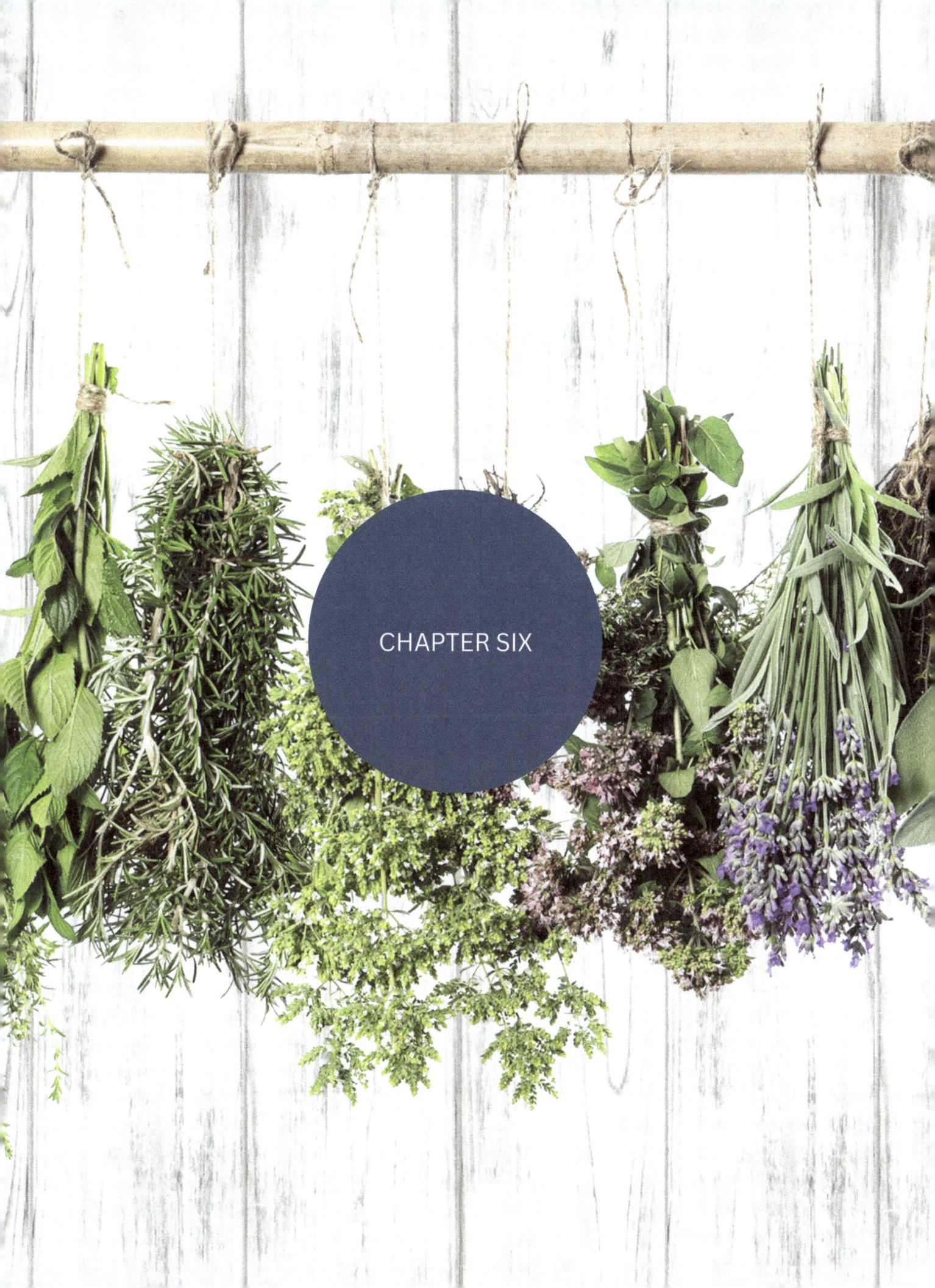

CHAPTER SIX

Latin American Herbal Traditions

Latin America is a treasure trove of medicinal plants and herbal traditions rooted in the diverse ecosystems of the Amazon rainforest, Andean highlands, and other rich landscapes. Indigenous knowledge, often passed through generations, forms the backbone of Latin American herbal medicine. These traditions integrate the spiritual, cultural, and therapeutic aspects of healing, reflecting the deep connection between people and nature.

Healing Practices from the Amazon and Beyond

The herbal traditions of Latin America are as varied as its geography. The Amazon rainforest alone is home to thousands of plant species with medicinal properties, many of which are yet to be fully studied. Across the region, herbal remedies are used not just to address physical ailments but also to harmonize the mind, body, and spirit.

1. Indigenous Wisdom and Spiritual Healing
    - Plants like ayahuasca and tobacco are used in spiritual ceremonies to cleanse the soul, remove negative energy, and connect with ancestral spirits.
    - Healing practices often include prayers, chants, and rituals, emphasizing the spiritual dimension of wellness.
2. Integration with Modern Medicine
    - Latin American herbal remedies have contributed to global pharmacology, with compounds like quinine and curare being adapted for modern medicine.
    - There is growing interest in studying these traditional practices to uncover new treatments for chronic and infectious diseases.

3. Sustainability and Conservation
    - With increasing demand for Amazonian herbs, sustainable harvesting practices are critical to preserving these plants for future generations.
    - Efforts are underway to protect indigenous knowledge and ensure fair trade for communities who cultivate and harvest these herbs.

Key Herbs and Their Uses
1. Chanca Piedra (Kidney Health)
    - Scientific Name: Phyllanthus niruri
    - Description: Known as the "stone breaker," chanca piedra is a powerful herb widely used to support kidney and urinary health.
    - Medicinal Uses:
        - Dissolves kidney stones and prevents their formation.
        - Treats urinary tract infections and promotes detoxification.
        - Supports liver health and aids digestion.
    - Preparation:
        - Leaves and stems are brewed into teas or decoctions.
        - Liquid extracts are used for concentrated doses.
2. Guarana (Energy Boost)
    - Scientific Name: Paullinia cupana
    - Description: A seed native to the Amazon, guarana is prized for its high caffeine content and ability to enhance energy and focus.
    - Medicinal Uses:
        - Provides a natural energy boost and fights fatigue.
        - Improves mental alertness and cognitive performance.
        - Acts as an appetite suppressant and supports weight management.

- **Preparation:**
  - Seeds are ground into powder and added to beverages.
  - Often included in energy drinks and herbal supplements.
3. **Yerba Mate (Cognitive Stimulant)**
   - **Scientific Name:** *Ilex paraguariensis*
   - **Description:** Yerba mate is a traditional beverage in South America, known for its energizing and social qualities.
   - **Medicinal Uses:**
     - Enhances mental clarity and concentration.
     - Supports digestion and metabolism.
     - Provides antioxidants and reduces inflammation.
   - **Preparation:**
     - Leaves are steeped in hot water and consumed as a tea, often shared socially in a gourd.
     - Can be blended with other herbs for added health benefits.
4. **Achiote (Annatto) (Anti-Inflammatory)**
   - **Scientific Name:** *Bixa orellana*
   - **Description:** Achiote seeds are known for their vibrant red color and medicinal properties, commonly used in Latin American cuisine and remedies.
   - **Medicinal Uses:**
     - Reduces inflammation and soothes skin conditions.
     - Supports digestive health and treats heartburn.
     - Acts as an antimicrobial agent for infections.
   - **Preparation:**
     - Seeds are infused in oil for topical applications.
     - Leaves are brewed into teas for internal use.

5. **Quinine (Malaria Treatment)**
    - **Scientific Name:** *Cinchona spp.*
    - **Description:** Extracted from the bark of the cinchona tree, quinine is one of the earliest treatments for malaria, a discovery rooted in Andean herbal traditions.
    - **Medicinal Uses:**
        - Treats malaria by killing the parasites in red blood cells.
        - Reduces fever and alleviates muscle pain.
        - Acts as a tonic for overall health improvement.
    - **Preparation:**
        - Bark is dried and ground into powder for medicinal use.
        - Quinine is now synthesized for pharmaceutical applications but remains a cornerstone of traditional medicine.

Latin American herbal traditions are a testament to the wisdom of indigenous communities and their ability to harness nature's healing power. These practices continue to inspire modern medicine while offering sustainable solutions for health and well-being.

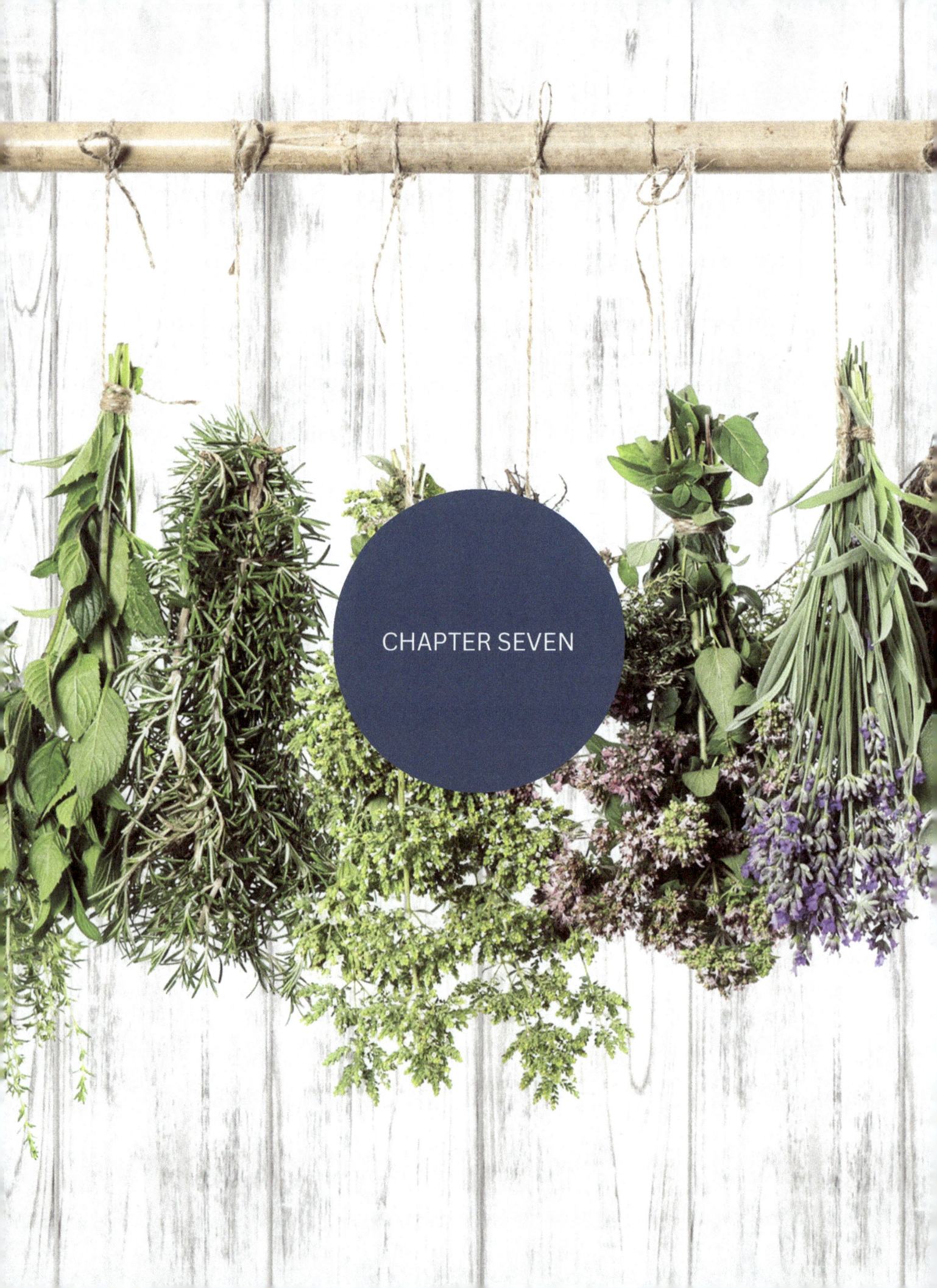

CHAPTER SEVEN

Oceanic and Polynesian Herbal Traditions

The herbal traditions of Oceanic and Polynesian cultures reflect the deep connection island communities have with their natural surroundings. Isolated by vast oceans, these cultures developed unique remedies that draw from the abundant resources of tropical rainforests, coastal flora, and volcanic soils. Traditional healers, known as kahunas in Polynesia or tohunga in Maori culture, played central roles in preserving and applying herbal knowledge for healing physical and spiritual ailments.

Healing Practices of Island Cultures

1. Integration of Spirituality and Medicine
   - Healing practices in Oceanic and Polynesian traditions often include spiritual elements such as chants, prayers, and rituals.
   - Herbs are used to harmonize the body and spirit, addressing imbalances believed to cause illness.
2. Sustainability in Herbal Gathering
   - Herbal traditions emphasize sustainable harvesting practices to ensure the preservation of native plants for future generations.
   - The natural environment is seen as sacred, and respectful gathering is considered essential to maintaining balance with nature.
3. Holistic Approaches to Wellness
   - Treatments often combine herbal remedies with physical therapies like massage (lomilomi) and steaming.
   - Diet and lifestyle adjustments are integral to the healing process.

Key Herbs and Their Uses

1. Kava (Stress and Anxiety Relief)
   - Scientific Name: Piper methysticum
   - Description: A traditional Polynesian plant, kava is known for its calming effects on the mind and body. It is prepared as a ceremonial beverage and consumed socially for relaxation.
   - Medicinal Uses:
     - Reduces stress and anxiety by acting on the central nervous system.
     - Promotes restful sleep and alleviates symptoms of insomnia.
     - Provides muscle relaxation and eases tension.
   - Preparation:
     - The roots are dried and ground into powder, then mixed with water to create a drink.
     - Capsules and extracts are also available for convenience.

2. Noni (Immunity and Skin Health)
   - Scientific Name: Morinda citrifolia
   - Description: Noni is a fruit-bearing tree native to the Pacific Islands. Its fruit, leaves, and roots are all used in traditional medicine.
   - Medicinal Uses:
     - Strengthens the immune system with its high antioxidant content.
     - Treats skin conditions like wounds, burns, and infections.
     - Improves digestion and supports joint health.
   - Preparation:
     - The fruit is fermented to produce juice, a common medicinal form.
     - Leaves are applied topically or brewed into teas.

3. Breadfruit Leaves (Diabetes Support)
    - Scientific Name: Artocarpus altilis
    - Description: Breadfruit is a staple food in many Oceanic diets, and its leaves have been used for centuries in traditional medicine.
    - Medicinal Uses:
        - Regulates blood sugar levels, making it beneficial for managing diabetes.
        - Acts as a diuretic to support kidney function.
        - Alleviates high blood pressure and promotes heart health.
    - Preparation:
        - Leaves are boiled to make teas or infusions.
        - Topical preparations are used for skin issues and wound care.

Oceanic and Polynesian herbal traditions exemplify a harmonious blend of culture, nature, and medicine. These practices remain vital in their communities and are gaining recognition for their therapeutic potential in modern medicine.

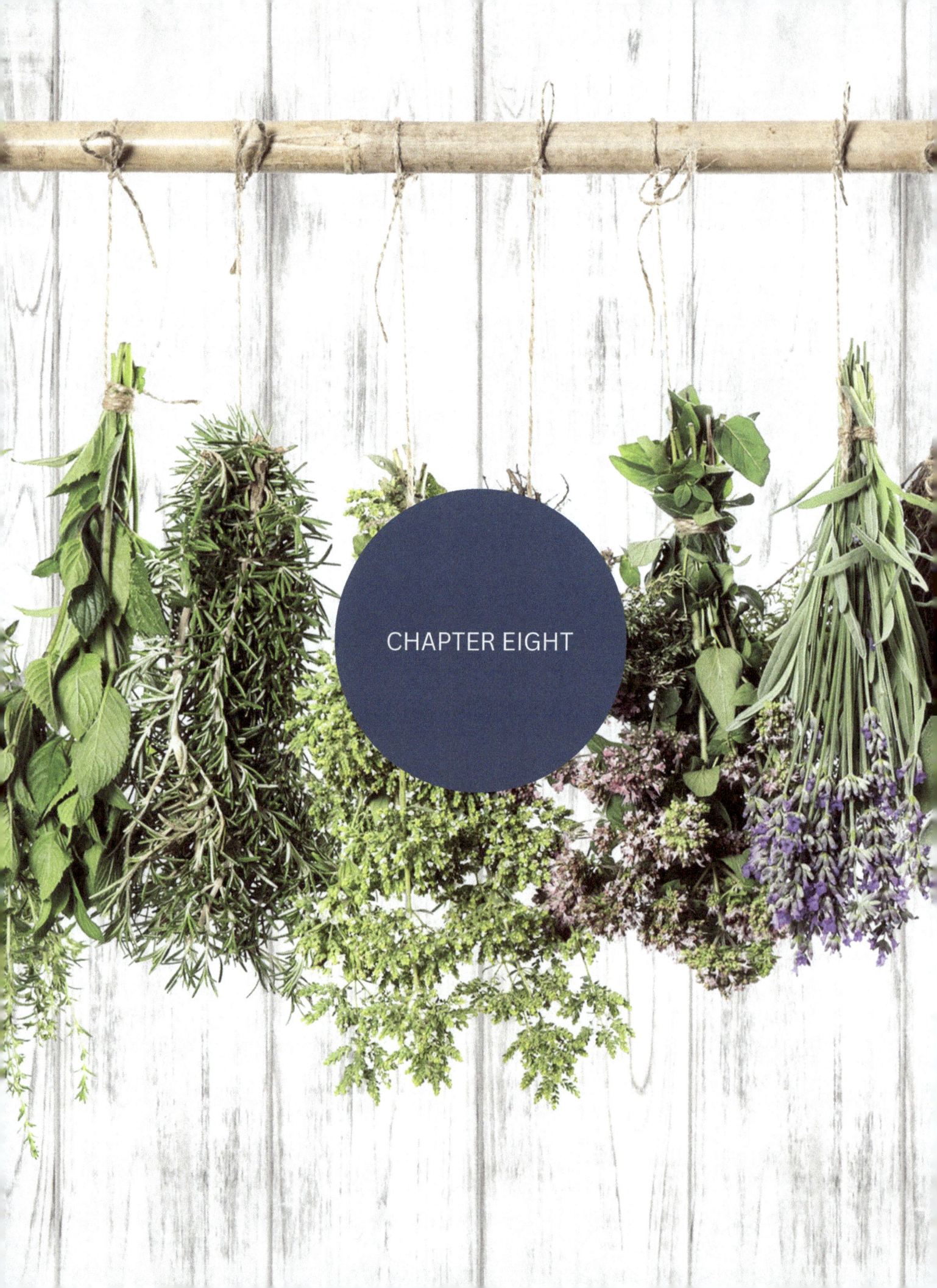

CHAPTER EIGHT

Crafting Herbal Remedies

Herbal remedies offer a natural approach to health and wellness, and crafting them at home allows for personalization and control over ingredients. This chapter focuses on essential techniques for beginners, guiding readers through the preparation of herbal teas, infusions, decoctions, tinctures, oils, and salves. These foundational methods form the backbone of herbal medicine, making it accessible to anyone interested in self-care with herbs.

Basic Preparations for Beginners

Crafting herbal remedies involves selecting the right herbs, preparing them correctly, and storing them to retain potency. Begin with fresh or dried herbs and use high-quality equipment to ensure effectiveness and safety.

1. Key Tools and Materials:
   - Non-reactive pots (stainless steel or glass).
   - Mortar and pestle for grinding herbs.
   - Measuring spoons and scales for accurate dosing.
   - Glass jars and bottles for storage.
   - Fine mesh strainers or cheesecloth for filtering.
2. Choosing the Right Herbs:
   - Start with well-known and safe herbs such as chamomile, peppermint, or calendula.
   - Research the properties of herbs to match remedies with desired outcomes.
3. Safety Tips:
   - Always test for allergic reactions before using a new herb.
   - Use recommended dosages and consult with a healthcare professional if needed.

Teas, Infusions, and Decoctions
1. Herbal Teas
    - Purpose: A quick and simple method for consuming herbs, often for mild ailments or daily wellness.
    - Preparation:
        - Add 1-2 teaspoons of dried herbs (or 2-3 teaspoons of fresh herbs) per cup of boiling water.
        - Steep for 5-10 minutes, strain, and enjoy.
    - Common Uses:
        - Chamomile tea for relaxation.
        - Peppermint tea for digestion.
2. Infusions
    - Purpose: Used to extract nutrients and medicinal compounds from delicate plant parts like leaves and flowers.
    - Preparation:
        - Use 1 ounce of dried herbs per quart of boiling water.
        - Cover and steep for 4-8 hours for maximum potency.
        - Strain and refrigerate for up to 2 days.
    - Common Uses:
        - Nettle infusion for energy and iron supplementation.
3. Decoctions
    - Purpose: Ideal for tougher plant parts like roots, bark, and seeds, which require prolonged simmering to release active compounds.
    - Preparation:
        - Use 1 ounce of dried herbs per quart of water.
        - Simmer gently for 20-40 minutes, then strain.
    - Common Uses:
        - Ginger root decoction for nausea and inflammation.
        - Cinnamon bark decoction for blood sugar regulation.

Tinctures, Oils, and Salves

1. **Tinctures**
   - Purpose: Concentrated herbal extracts made with alcohol or glycerin, used for long-term storage and convenience.
   - Preparation:
     - Fill a jar with dried herbs and cover with alcohol (vodka or brandy) at a 1:5 ratio (herb:solvent).
     - Seal and shake daily, allowing it to steep for 4-6 weeks.
     - Strain and bottle the liquid in dropper bottles.
   - Common Uses:
     - Echinacea tincture for immune support.
     - Valerian root tincture for sleep aid.

2. **Herbal Oils**
   - Purpose: Used for massage, skincare, or as a base for salves.
   - Preparation:
     - Combine dried herbs and a carrier oil (e.g., olive or almond oil) in a jar.
     - Steep in sunlight for 2-3 weeks or use a slow cooker on the lowest setting for 4-6 hours.
     - Strain and store in a dark, cool place.
   - Common Uses:
     - Calendula oil for soothing skin irritations.
     - Arnica oil for sore muscles and bruises.

3. **Herbal Salves**
   - Purpose: Healing balms made by combining herbal oils with beeswax for topical application.
   - Preparation:
     - Melt 1 ounce of beeswax with 4 ounces of herbal oil in a double boiler.
     - Stir, pour into tins, and let it cool and solidify.
   - Common Uses:
     - Comfrey salve for wound healing.
     - Tea tree salve for antibacterial protection.

Advanced Techniques in Crafting Herbal Remedies

Once you've mastered the basics of crafting herbal remedies, you may want to explore more advanced techniques that can enhance the potency and versatility of your herbal preparations. This chapter focuses on creating herbal capsules and powders, as well as crafting herbal ferments and tonics. These methods are particularly useful for those looking to use herbs in a more concentrated form or for long-term health benefits.

Making Herbal Capsules and Powders

1. Herbal Powders
   - Purpose: Herbal powders are concentrated, dried, and finely ground herbs that can be used in a variety of ways, such as in capsules, teas, or added to food and smoothies.
   - Preparation:
     - Choosing Herbs: Use herbs that are naturally dense in medicinal compounds, such as turmeric, ginger, or ashwagandha.
     - Drying: Ensure herbs are properly dried before grinding to prevent mold growth. Air-drying or dehydrating herbs works best.
     - Grinding: Use a mortar and pestle, spice grinder, or coffee grinder to grind dried herbs into a fine powder.
     - Storage: Store powders in airtight containers, preferably glass jars, in a cool, dark place. Powdered herbs can lose potency if exposed to light or heat for long periods.
   - Common Uses:
     - Turmeric powder for anti-inflammatory benefits.
     - Ashwagandha powder for stress reduction and adrenal support.
     - Spirulina powder for nutrient-dense boosts.

1. Making Herbal Capsules
    - Purpose: Herbal capsules allow for precise, convenient, and portable dosing. This is a great way to take herbs daily without the taste or preparation time associated with teas or tinctures.
    - Preparation:
        - Ingredients: Choose herbs in powdered form, such as powdered ginger, echinacea, or ginseng.
        - Capsule Size: Empty vegetable capsules (typically size 00) can be purchased online or at health food stores.
        - Filling the Capsules:
            - Use a capsule filling machine for ease and consistency (available for small batches).
            - Simply fill the capsules with the powdered herb, being careful to pack the powder evenly to prevent air pockets.
        - Storage: Store filled capsules in airtight containers in a cool, dry place.
        - Dosage: It is essential to adhere to dosage recommendations to ensure safety and effectiveness. A typical dosage is 1-2 capsules per day for general health support, but specific herbs may vary.
    - Common Uses:
        - Ashwagandha for stress management.
        - Rhodiola for energy and endurance.
        - Garlic powder for cardiovascular health.

Crafting Herbal Ferments and Tonics

1. Herbal Tonics
    - Purpose: Herbal tonics are liquid preparations made by infusing or decocting herbs, often combined with other ingredients like honey, vinegar, or apple cider vinegar. They are typically consumed to promote general wellness and provide long-lasting health benefits.
    - Preparation:
        - Ingredients: Common tonic ingredients include ginger, garlic, cayenne pepper, and honey, each contributing to digestion, circulation, or immunity.
        - Infusion Method: To make a tonic, combine herbs (fresh or dried) with water or vinegar and steep them for 4-6 weeks. For quicker results, you can simmer the herbs in water for a more potent decoction.
        - Storage: Store the tonic in glass jars or bottles, preferably dark-colored to protect from light.
        - Usage: Herbal tonics are often taken 1-2 tablespoons daily to support overall health.
    - Common Uses:
        - Apple cider vinegar tonic with garlic and ginger for digestive health.
        - Turmeric and black pepper tonic for inflammation.
2. Crafting Herbal Ferments
    - Purpose: Herbal ferments combine the medicinal benefits of herbs with the probiotic power of fermentation. Fermented herbal preparations can help with gut health, digestion, and immune support.

- Preparation:
  - Ingredients: Common herbs used in fermentation include ginger, mint, dandelion root, and chamomile.
  - Fermentation Process:
    - Place fresh or dried herbs in a jar and cover them with a liquid like water or herbal tea.
    - Add a fermentation starter such as whey, kefir grains, or a bit of raw apple cider vinegar to kickstart the process.
    - Seal the jar tightly and allow it to ferment at room temperature for 3-7 days, checking daily.
  - Straining and Bottling: Once the desired fermentation is achieved, strain out the herbs, and bottle the liquid.
- Storage: Fermented herbal drinks should be stored in the refrigerator once the fermentation process is complete.
- Common Uses:
  - Ginger kombucha for digestive health.
  - Dandelion root fermented tonic for liver detox.
  - Chamomile and lavender fermented tonic for relaxation.

Benefits of Advanced Herbal Preparations
1. Potency and Concentration
   - Advanced methods like capsules, powders, and tonics often concentrate the beneficial compounds in herbs, making them more potent and effective for therapeutic use.
   - These forms allow for long-term storage and easy use in everyday routines.
2. Customization
   - By crafting your own remedies, you can tailor herbal preparations to your specific needs and preferences. Whether you need energy, immunity, stress relief, or digestive support, these techniques enable you to create personalized health solutions.

1. **Increased Bioavailability**
   - Some advanced preparations, like tinctures and ferments, can increase the bioavailability of certain herbal compounds, helping your body absorb and utilize them more effectively.

As you gain experience, crafting more advanced herbal remedies will become an integral part of your natural health practice. These techniques offer flexibility, potency, and ease of use, making them ideal for both personal wellness and creating herbal remedies to share with others. Would you like to delve further into the preparation of specific tonics or ferments?

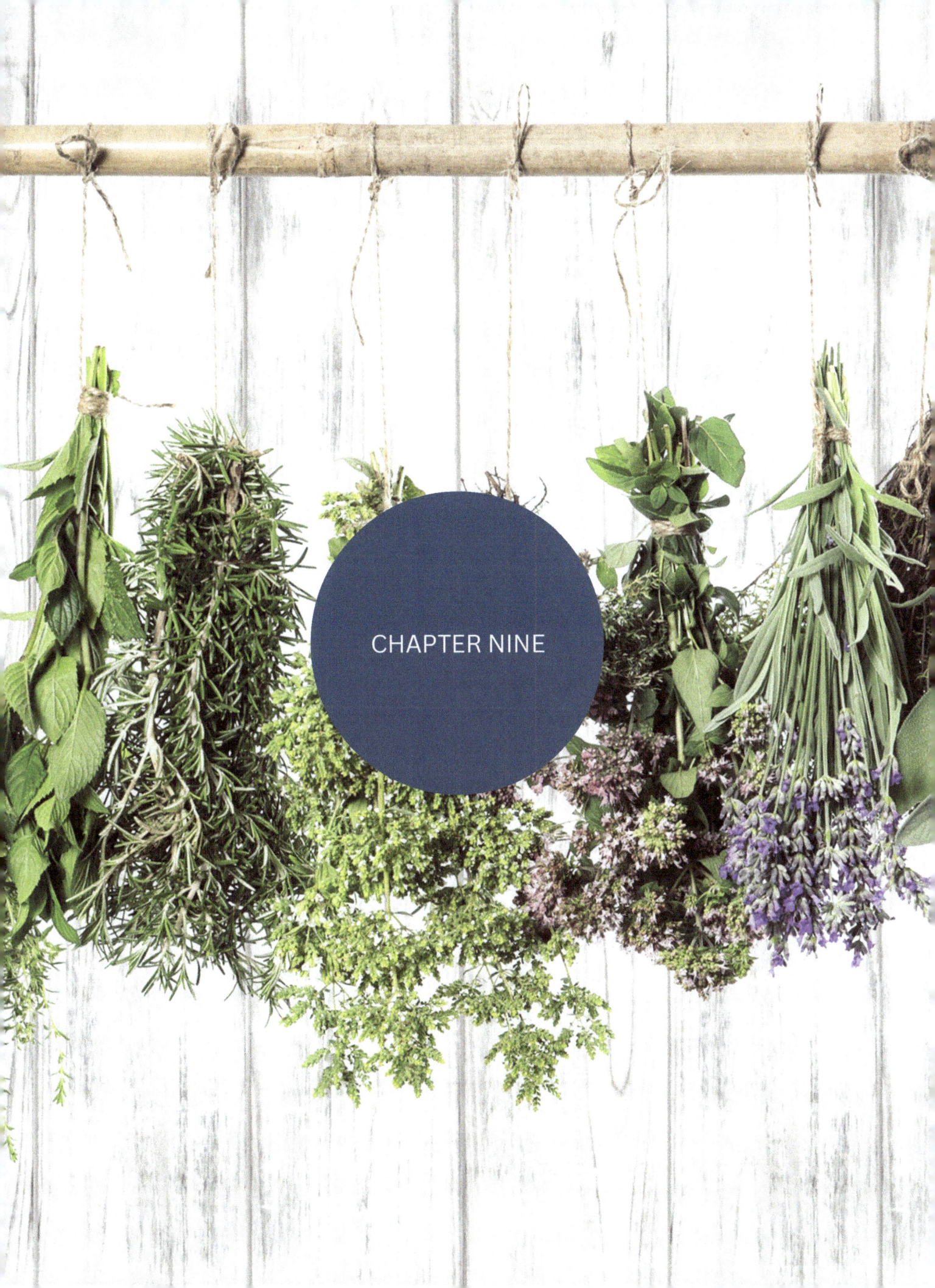

CHAPTER NINE

Essential Oils from Every Continent

Aromatherapy, the practice of using essential oils for therapeutic purposes, is an ancient healing tradition that spans cultures and continents. The essential oils derived from plants have been used for centuries to treat physical and emotional ailments, promote relaxation, and enhance overall well-being. In this chapter, we explore essential oils from around the world and how to blend them effectively for health and wellness.

Essential Oils from Every Continent
1. Africa: Nature's Rich Aromatics
2. Africa is home to a wide variety of aromatic plants, many of which are used in traditional healing practices. African essential oils are known for their potency, diverse therapeutic properties, and vibrant scents.
    - Frankincense (Boswellia carterii):
        - Benefits: Known for its grounding properties, frankincense oil is excellent for reducing stress and anxiety, promoting relaxation, and supporting respiratory health.
        - Use: Often used in meditation and spiritual practices, it is also an excellent oil for skincare and promoting healthy skin regeneration.
    - Rooibos (Aspalathus linearis):
        - Benefits: Rooibos is widely known for its antioxidant and anti-inflammatory properties. The essential oil is helpful in calming the skin, reducing redness, and promoting relaxation.
        - Use: It is ideal for skin irritations and can be blended into carrier oils for soothing body massages.
    - Lemongrass (Cymbopogon citratus):
        - Benefits: Lemongrass oil has antimicrobial properties and is widely used to reduce inflammation and fight infections. It is also excellent for stimulating the immune system and enhancing circulation.

- **Use**: Best for use in cleaning products, massage oils, or diffusers to uplift mood and clear the mind.

1. **Asia: Ancient Healing with Aromatic Herbs**
2. Asia has a long history of using plant-based remedies, and essential oils from this region are treasured for their healing properties in both traditional medicine and modern wellness practices.
    - **Sandalwood (Santalum album)**:
        - **Benefits**: Sandalwood is known for its calming and grounding effects. It is often used in aromatherapy for meditation, stress relief, and enhancing emotional clarity.
        - **Use**: Ideal for creating peaceful environments, this oil also has moisturizing properties for dry skin and can be used in anti-aging skincare formulations.
    - **Tea Tree (Melaleuca alternifolia)**:
        - **Benefits**: Native to Australia but widely used in Asian traditions, tea tree oil is one of the most powerful antibacterial and antifungal oils. It is ideal for treating skin issues such as acne, fungal infections, and wounds.
        - **Use**: Tea tree oil can be diluted in carrier oils for topical application or used in a diffuser to purify the air.
    - **Jasmine (Jasminum sambac)**:
        - **Benefits**: Jasmine essential oil is known for its antidepressant and aphrodisiac qualities. It can help to boost mood, alleviate anxiety, and promote emotional balance.
        - **Use**: Often used in perfumery, it can also be used in massage oils to relieve muscle tension and emotional stress.

1. **Europe: Refined and Calming Oils**
2. Europe has contributed some of the most well-known essential oils, many of which have become staples in aromatherapy practices around the world. The oils from this region are often used for both physical and emotional healing.
    - **Lavender (Lavandula angustifolia)**:
        - **Benefits**: Lavender is one of the most versatile essential oils, known for its calming and healing properties. It is used to alleviate stress, improve sleep, and reduce pain.
        - **Use**: It can be diffused to create a calming atmosphere, applied topically for skin care, or used in a warm bath for a relaxing experience.
    - **Rose (Rosa damascena)**:
        - **Benefits**: Rose oil is considered one of the most therapeutic oils for emotional healing. It is excellent for reducing symptoms of depression, anxiety, and stress while promoting emotional stability.
        - **Use**: Frequently used in skincare for its anti-aging and skin-healing properties, it can be added to face creams or used in massage blends.
    - **Peppermint (Mentha piperita)**:
        - **Benefits**: Peppermint oil has a cooling effect and is often used to alleviate headaches, migraines, and muscle pain. It also has energizing properties and helps clear the mind.
        - **Use**: Best for use in blends designed to refresh and energize, as well as for digestive support.

1. **The Americas: Plant Remedies with Ancient Wisdom**
2. The Americas, particularly through the indigenous cultures of North and South America, have a wealth of knowledge regarding plant-based remedies. Essential oils from this region have been gaining popularity for their ability to provide natural relief for various conditions.
    - **Cedarwood (Cedrus atlantica)**:
        - **Benefits**: Cedarwood essential oil has grounding and calming properties. It is used to promote restful sleep, clear respiratory pathways, and reduce stress.
        - **Use**: Commonly used in meditation, as well as in products designed to relieve coughs and colds.
    - **Sweet Orange (Citrus sinensis)**:
        - **Benefits**: Sweet orange oil is uplifting and invigorating. It is known to boost mood, improve digestion, and act as a mild sedative for anxiety.
        - **Use**: Best used in diffusers to create a cheerful, positive atmosphere or in bath oils for a soothing and revitalizing experience.
    - **Palo Santo (Bursera graveolens)**:
        - **Benefits**: Native to the Amazon rainforest, Palo Santo is used to purify the air, clear negative energy, and alleviate stress.
        - **Use**: This oil is commonly burned in rituals or used in diffusers for relaxation and spiritual cleansing.

Oceania: Unique and Soothing Oils

1. Oceania, particularly the Pacific Islands, is known for its distinctive, soothing essential oils. These oils are integral to the cultures of the islands, where they are used for a variety of therapeutic purposes.
    - **Kava (Piper methysticum)**:
        - **Benefits**: Kava root essential oil is renowned for its ability to reduce anxiety, promote relaxation, and relieve muscle tension.
        - **Use**: Often used for stress relief and relaxation, Kava oil can be applied topically or diffused to create a calm atmosphere.
    - **Manuka (Leptospermum scoparium)**:
        - **Benefits**: Manuka oil is known for its antibacterial and healing properties. It is used for skin conditions, wound healing, and as a natural remedy for colds and respiratory issues.
        - **Use**: Ideal for use in skincare products, as well as in teas or steam inhalations for respiratory health.

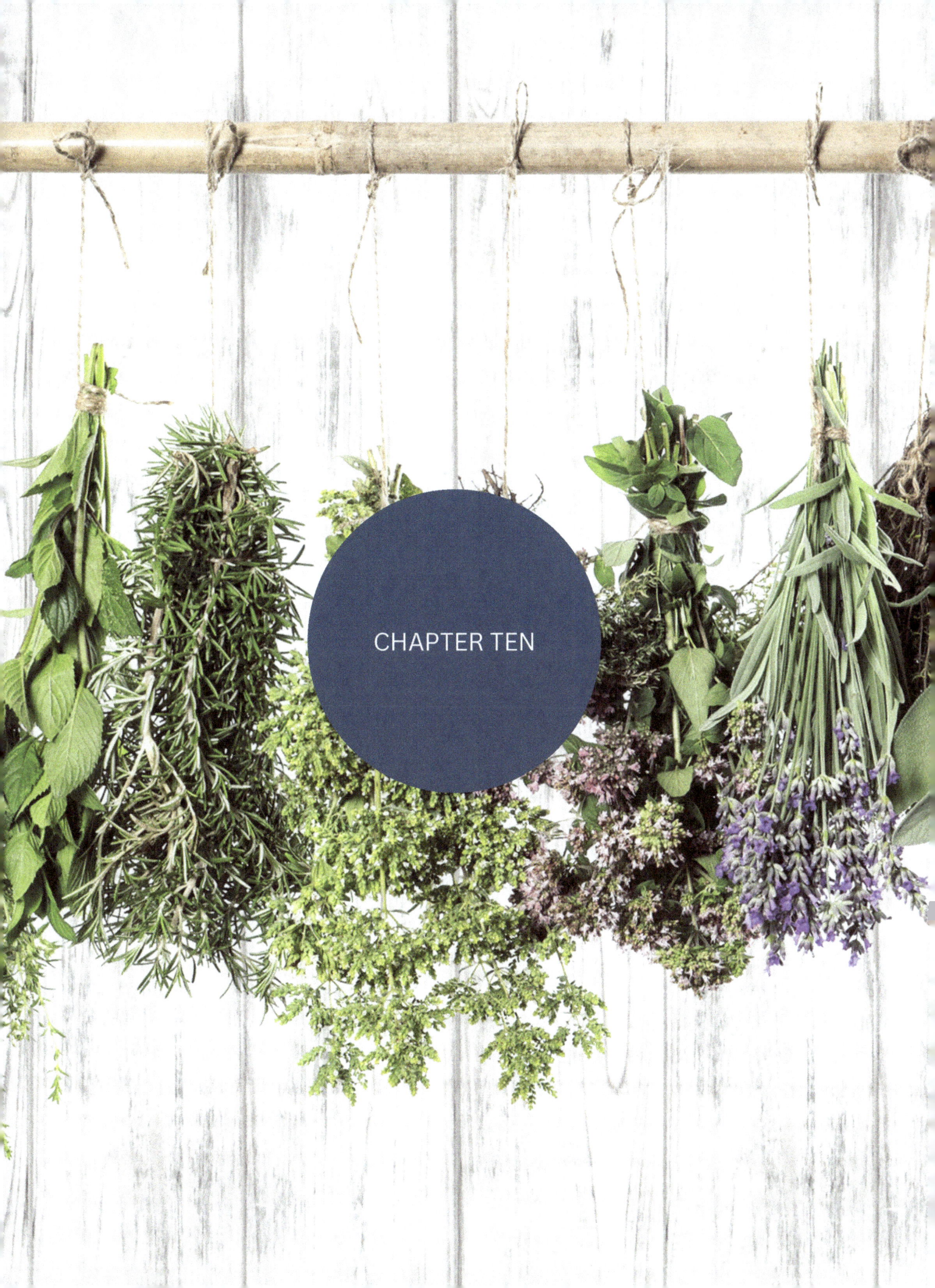

CHAPTER TEN

Blending for Health and Wellness

Blending essential oils is an art, and when done correctly, it can provide powerful healing effects that go beyond the individual benefits of each oil. Understanding the proper ratios and blending methods can help you create personalized remedies that target specific health concerns.

1. Basic Blending Principles
    - Top, Middle, and Base Notes:
        - Top Notes: These are the lightest oils that evaporate quickly and create the first impression of a blend. Examples: citrus oils (e.g., lemon, orange), eucalyptus, peppermint.
        - Middle Notes: These oils are often referred to as the "heart" of the blend and have a moderate evaporation rate. Examples: lavender, geranium, rosemary.
        - Base Notes: These oils have the longest-lasting scent and provide depth to the blend. Examples: sandalwood, cedarwood, frankincense.
    - Blending for Therapeutic Purposes:
        - Stress Relief: Combine lavender (middle note), frankincense (base note), and sweet orange (top note) for a calming and grounding blend.
        - Energy Boost: A blend of peppermint (top note), lemon (top note), and rosemary (middle note) can help invigorate the mind and body.
    - Dilution: Always dilute essential oils before topical use. A standard dilution ratio is 2-5 drops of essential oil per tablespoon of carrier oil for adults, and less for children or sensitive skin.
2. Essential Oil Diffusion
    - Diffuser Blends: Create specific blends depending on your goal (e.g., relaxation, focus, energy) and add them to an ultrasonic or nebulizing diffuser.
    - Room Sprays: Mix essential oils with water and a small amount of alcohol or witch hazel to create a spray for freshening rooms or linen.

Topical Applications
- **Massage Oils**: Create a calming blend using lavender, chamomile, and ylang-ylang to help reduce stress and promote relaxation.
- **Skincare Oils**: For anti-aging or acne-prone skin, combine tea tree oil with lavender and rosehip oil.

Aromatherapy offers a unique and holistic approach to health and wellness, using the potent healing properties of essential oils from around the world. By blending oils from different continents, you can harness the diverse and rich traditions of plant medicine to create effective, natural remedies tailored to your individual needs.

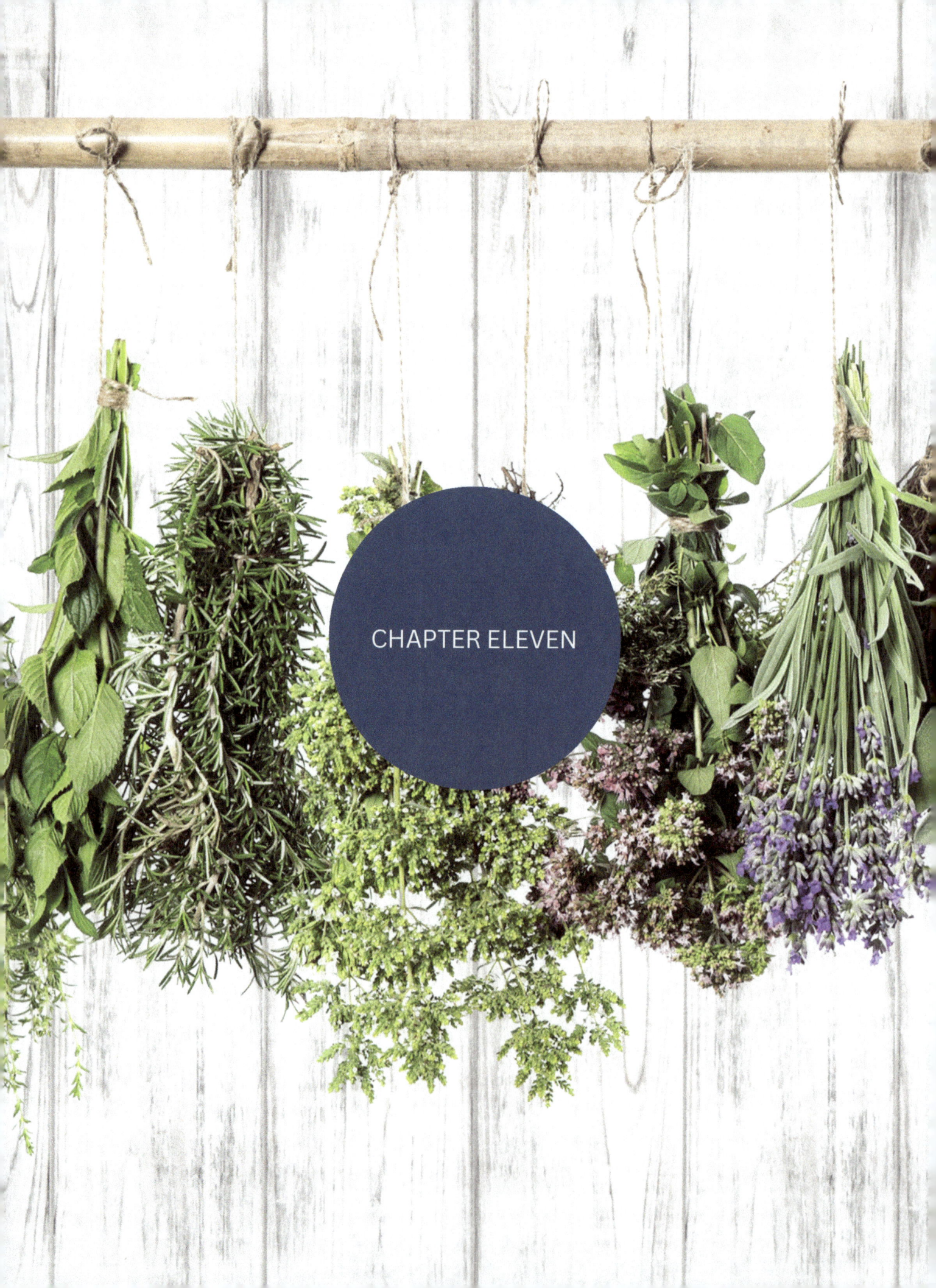

CHAPTER ELEVEN

Building Your Herbal First Aid Kit: Remedies for Cuts, Bruises, and Infections

A well-stocked herbal first aid kit is a vital tool for any home, especially for those who want to rely on natural remedies to address common injuries and ailments. While it's important to understand the basics of using herbal remedies, it's also crucial to recognize when medical attention is necessary. This chapter will guide you through the essential herbs to include in your first aid kit and how to use them effectively for cuts, bruises, and infections.

Essential Herbs for Your Herbal First Aid Kit
1. Calendula (Calendula officinalis)
    - Uses: Calendula is a powerful herb for skin healing, widely used in creams, oils, and tinctures for its anti-inflammatory, antibacterial, and antifungal properties. It is ideal for treating cuts, abrasions, burns, and bruises.
    - How to Use: Apply calendula ointment or cream directly to cuts and scrapes to promote faster healing. It can also be used as a poultice for deeper wounds, helping to prevent infection and reduce swelling.
    - Preparation: For a soothing infusion, steep dried calendula flowers in hot water for 10-15 minutes. Use as a rinse for cuts or as a compress for bruises.

1. **Comfrey (Symphytum officinale)**
   - **Uses**: Known as the "knitbone" herb, comfrey is highly regarded for its ability to speed up the healing of bones, muscles, and connective tissues. It's ideal for bruises, sprains, and broken skin.
   - **How to Use**: Apply a comfrey salve or poultice to bruises or sprains to reduce inflammation and promote faster healing of the tissue. Comfrey can also be used for joint pain relief.
   - **Preparation**: To make a poultice, crush fresh comfrey leaves and apply directly to the injured area, securing with a bandage. Alternatively, use comfrey oil or salve for a gentler application.
2. **Plantain (Plantago major)**
   - **Uses**: Plantain is a versatile herb often used for its wound-healing and anti-inflammatory properties. It helps with stopping bleeding, soothing skin irritation, and reducing swelling.
   - **How to Use**: Apply fresh plantain leaves directly to cuts or insect bites to stop bleeding and prevent infection. The leaves are also great for reducing swelling and promoting the regeneration of damaged tissue.
   - **Preparation**: For a poultice, crush fresh plantain leaves and apply to the affected area. For cuts, simply place the fresh leaves over the wound and secure them with a bandage.
3. **Lavender (Lavandula angustifolia)**
   - **Uses**: Lavender oil is widely known for its calming and antiseptic properties, making it effective for treating burns, cuts, and infections. It also helps to prevent scarring.
   - **How to Use**: Apply diluted lavender essential oil directly to cuts, burns, or bruises. It works to relieve pain and discomfort, while its antiseptic properties prevent infection.
   - **Preparation**: Mix a few drops of lavender essential oil with a carrier oil, such as coconut or olive oil, before applying it to the affected area. For burns, a few drops of lavender essential oil mixed in cool water can help soothe the skin.

4. **Yarrow (Achillea millefolium)**
   - **Uses**: Yarrow is an herb with a long history of use in wound care. It has antiseptic, anti-inflammatory, and astringent properties that make it excellent for stopping bleeding, healing wounds, and preventing infections.
   - **How to Use**: Yarrow can be used to stop bleeding and promote healing in cuts and abrasions. It can also help with bruises by reducing swelling and alleviating pain.
   - **Preparation**: Apply yarrow tincture or powder to the cut or wound to stop bleeding. You can also create a poultice by crushing fresh yarrow leaves and applying them to the affected area.

5. **Tea Tree Oil (Melaleuca alternifolia)**
   - **Uses**: Tea tree oil is a potent antiseptic and antibacterial agent, making it effective for treating cuts, scrapes, and infections. It's commonly used in natural first aid kits for its ability to clean and disinfect.
   - **How to Use**: Dilute tea tree oil with a carrier oil and apply to cuts, bruises, or infected areas to help cleanse the wound and prevent bacterial growth.
   - **Preparation**: A few drops of tea tree oil mixed with a tablespoon of carrier oil can be used as a topical application for treating wounds.

Remedies for Cuts, Bruises, and Infections

1. For Cuts and Scrapes:
   - Step 1: Clean the wound with water and mild soap. Avoid using harsh chemicals that can irritate the skin.
   - Step 2: Apply a disinfecting herbal remedy such as tea tree oil, lavender oil, or yarrow to prevent infection. Dilute essential oils with a carrier oil to avoid irritation.
   - Step 3: If the wound is still open and bleeding, apply plantain leaves or yarrow to help stop the bleeding.
   - Step 4: Cover the wound with a sterile bandage and replace it with fresh herbs or ointment as necessary.
2. For Bruises:
   - Step 1: Apply a cold compress or ice pack to the bruised area immediately to reduce swelling and inflammation.
   - Step 2: After 24 hours, apply a herbal salve made from comfrey or arnica to promote healing and reduce bruising.
   - Step 3: For deep bruises, use a calendula infusion or oil for its anti-inflammatory properties to soothe the area.
3. For Infections:
   - Step 1: Use tea tree oil or lavender oil as a natural antiseptic to cleanse the area around the infection.
   - Step 2: For an internal infection, echinacea or garlic may help boost the immune system. Drink an infusion of echinacea or take garlic capsules or fresh garlic for its antimicrobial properties.
   - Step 3: Apply manuka honey directly to the infection. Manuka honey has potent antibacterial properties and is particularly effective for healing wounds and preventing infection.

Creating Herbal Poultices for Immediate Relief

Herbal poultices are simple to make and can provide quick relief for injuries, cuts, bruises, and infections. Here's how to create one:

1. For a Bruise:
    - Ingredients: Fresh comfrey or arnica leaves, cabbage leaves (optional for cooling effect).
    - Method: Crush the fresh herbs (or chop them) and mix them with a small amount of warm water to create a paste. Apply directly to the bruised area and cover with a bandage.
2. For a Cut or Scrape:
    - Ingredients: Fresh plantain leaves or yarrow.
    - Method: Crush the leaves to release their juices and apply directly to the wound. Secure the poultice with a clean bandage and replace it with fresh herbs as needed.

Essential Oils for First Aid Kit

In addition to herbal tinctures and salves, essential oils can provide quick remedies for various ailments. Include the following oils in your first aid kit:

- Lavender Oil: For burns, cuts, and stress relief.
- Tea Tree Oil: For infections and wound care.
- Peppermint Oil: For pain relief and cooling burns or headaches.
- Eucalyptus Oil: For respiratory infections, coughs, and muscle pain.
- Chamomile Oil: For calming irritated skin, inflammation, and wound healing.

A well-curated herbal first aid kit can serve as an invaluable tool for addressing common injuries and ailments using the power of nature. By learning how to prepare and use these herbs and remedies, you can address cuts, bruises, and infections effectively, without relying on synthetic chemicals. The herbs and remedies in your kit should be seen as part of a holistic approach to health, always complemented by common-sense practices, such as cleaning wounds properly and seeking professional medical care when necessary. With the right herbs on hand, you can confidently manage minor injuries and support your body's healing process naturally.

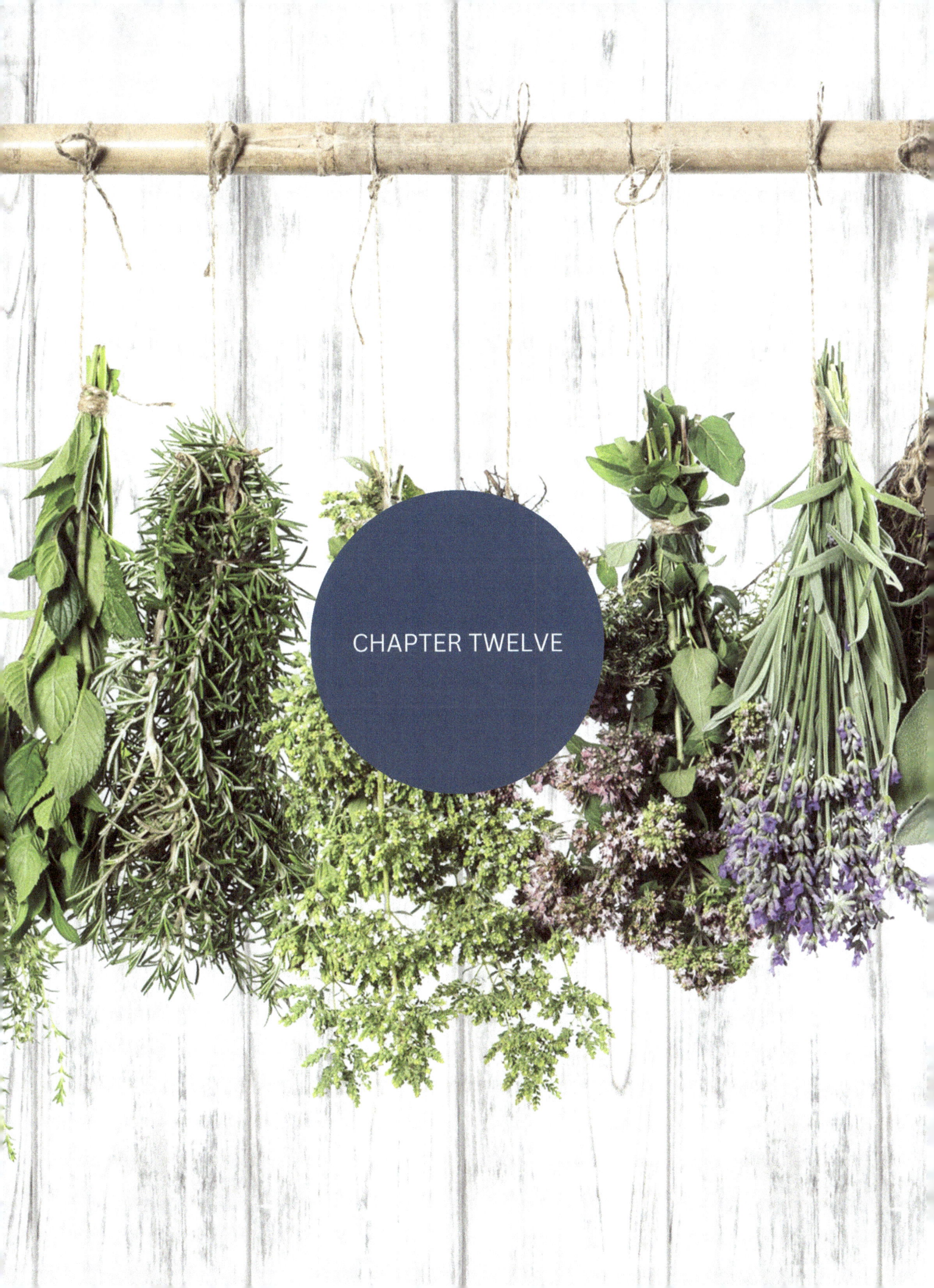

CHAPTER TWELVE

Remedies for Common Ailments

Herbal remedies have been used for centuries to address common ailments, supporting the body's natural healing processes. Whether you're battling a cold, digestive discomfort, stress, or skin issues, the right herbs can offer effective, natural relief. In this section, we'll explore some of the most powerful herbs and remedies for common health problems, including immune support, digestive health, stress and anxiety relief, and skin care.

Immune Support: Colds, Flu, and Allergies

A strong immune system is essential for protecting the body against infections like colds, the flu, and allergies. These herbs are well-known for their immune-boosting properties:

1. Echinacea (Echinacea purpurea)
    - Uses: Echinacea is one of the most popular herbs for boosting immune function. It can help reduce the severity and duration of colds and flu.
    - How to Use: Take as a tea, tincture, or capsule at the first sign of a cold or infection. Echinacea works best when used at the onset of symptoms.
    - Preparation: Brew echinacea tea from dried flowers or use a tincture. It's commonly used in combination with other immune-boosting herbs like elderberry.
2. Elderberry (Sambucus nigra)
    - Uses: Elderberry has antiviral properties and is commonly used to fight colds, the flu, and other viral infections.
    - How to Use: Elderberry syrup is a popular remedy for viral infections. It can also be taken as a tea or in capsule form.
    - Preparation: Elderberry syrup can be made at home by simmering elderberries with water, honey, and spices like cinnamon and cloves.

3. **Ginger (Zingiber officinale)**
    - **Uses**: Ginger is known for its ability to fight inflammation, ease congestion, and help with nausea.
    - **How to Use**: Drink ginger tea to reduce symptoms of cold, flu, and sore throat. You can also use fresh ginger root in hot water with honey and lemon for added benefits.
    - **Preparation**: Slice fresh ginger root and steep it in boiling water for about 10 minutes. Add honey and lemon for soothing effects.
4. **Astragalus (Astragalus membranaceus)**
    - **Uses**: Astragalus is a traditional herb used to enhance immune function and improve resistance to colds and infections.
    - **How to Use**: Take as a tincture, tea, or supplement. It's often used as a preventive remedy to strengthen the immune system over time.
    - **Preparation**: Use astragalus root in a decoction or as part of an herbal immune blend.
5. **Peppermint (Mentha piperita)**
    - **Uses**: Peppermint is a great herb for relieving respiratory symptoms, including sinus congestion, and for soothing sore throats.
    - **How to Use**: Drink peppermint tea or inhale steam from peppermint oil to help clear nasal passages.
    - **Preparation**: Brew peppermint tea by steeping fresh or dried leaves in hot water. You can also add a few drops of peppermint essential oil to a bowl of steaming water and inhale the vapor.

Digestive Health: Bloating, Nausea, Constipation

Herbs have long been used to soothe digestive issues and support gut health. Here are some herbs that can help alleviate common digestive problems:

1. Peppermint (Mentha piperita)
    - Uses: Peppermint is excellent for soothing digestive issues such as bloating, gas, and nausea. It can also aid in relieving irritable bowel syndrome (IBS) symptoms.
    - How to Use: Drink peppermint tea or use peppermint essential oil to ease digestive discomfort.
    - Preparation: Make a simple peppermint tea by steeping a handful of fresh or dried peppermint leaves in hot water for 5-10 minutes.
2. Ginger (Zingiber officinale)
    - Uses: Ginger is renowned for its ability to ease nausea and reduce bloating and indigestion. It is also useful for easing motion sickness and nausea caused by pregnancy or chemotherapy.
    - How to Use: Drink ginger tea or take ginger supplements to relieve digestive discomfort.
    - Preparation: Steep fresh ginger slices in hot water for a soothing tea. You can also chew on a small piece of fresh ginger for immediate relief.
3. Fennel (Foeniculum vulgare)
    - Uses: Fennel helps reduce bloating, gas, and indigestion. It can also ease stomach cramps and improve digestion.
    - How to Use: Fennel seeds can be chewed after meals or made into a soothing tea to relieve bloating and discomfort.
    - Preparation: Steep fennel seeds in boiling water for 10-15 minutes to create a mild, soothing tea.

5. **Chamomile (Matricaria chamomilla)**
    - **Uses**: Chamomile is known for its ability to relax the digestive system and relieve symptoms of indigestion, bloating, and nausea.
    - **How to Use**: Drink chamomile tea to soothe digestive upset, especially before bedtime for its calming effects.
    - **Preparation**: Brew chamomile tea with dried flowers or buy pre-packaged chamomile tea bags for easy use.
6. **Slippery Elm (Ulmus rubra)**
    - **Uses**: Slippery elm is great for soothing inflammation in the digestive tract and providing relief from constipation, diarrhea, and indigestion.
    - **How to Use**: Take slippery elm in powder form mixed with warm water, or use it in herbal capsules.
    - **Preparation**: Mix slippery elm powder with water to form a gel-like consistency, then drink it to help soothe and heal the digestive tract.

Stress and Anxiety Relief

Many herbs are known for their calming effects on the nervous system, making them ideal for managing stress, anxiety, and sleep disturbances. Here are a few key herbs that help with relaxation and mental clarity:

1. Lavender (Lavandula angustifolia)
    - Uses: Lavender is one of the best-known herbs for stress relief, helping to reduce anxiety, promote relaxation, and improve sleep quality.
    - How to Use: Use lavender essential oil for aromatherapy, or drink lavender tea for its calming effects.
    - Preparation: Add a few drops of lavender oil to a diffuser or inhale it directly. Alternatively, brew a cup of lavender tea from dried flowers.
2. Ashwagandha (Withania somnifera)
    - Uses: Ashwagandha is an adaptogen that helps the body adapt to stress, reduces anxiety, and improves overall energy levels.
    - How to Use: Take as a tincture or capsule for general stress relief and mental clarity.
    - Preparation: Ashwagandha is commonly available in powder form. Mix it into a smoothie, tea, or warm milk.

3. **Chamomile (Matricaria chamomilla)**
   - **Uses**: Chamomile is well-known for its mild sedative properties, making it a great choice for alleviating stress and promoting restful sleep.
   - **How to Use**: Drink chamomile tea to unwind after a stressful day or use chamomile essential oil in a diffuser.
   - **Preparation**: Brew chamomile tea with dried flowers, or use a chamomile essential oil diffuser before bedtime.
4. **Holy Basil (Tulsi) (Ocimum sanctum)**
   - **Uses**: Holy basil, also known as tulsi, is an adaptogen that helps reduce stress, anxiety, and cortisol levels.
   - **How to Use**: Drink holy basil tea or take as a supplement to support your body during stressful times.
   - **Preparation**: Steep fresh or dried holy basil leaves in hot water to make a soothing tea.
5. **Lemon Balm (Melissa officinalis)**
   - **Uses**: Lemon balm has a mild sedative effect and can help alleviate stress, anxiety, and insomnia.
   - **How to Use**: Drink lemon balm tea or apply lemon balm essential oil to your temples for quick relief.
   - **Preparation**: Brew a cup of lemon balm tea from fresh or dried leaves, or diffuse the essential oil for relaxation.

Skin Health

Herbs have been used for centuries to treat a wide range of skin conditions, from acne to eczema and dry skin. These herbs can help improve skin health naturally:

1. Aloe Vera (Aloe barbadensis miller)
   - Uses: Aloe vera is renowned for its ability to soothe burns, heal wounds, and provide relief for dry or irritated skin.
   - How to Use: Apply fresh aloe vera gel to burns, rashes, or acne spots for immediate relief and healing.
   - Preparation: Extract fresh gel from the aloe vera plant and apply directly to the skin. You can also use aloe vera gel or juice in cosmetic products.
2. Calendula (Calendula officinalis)
   - Uses: Calendula is a great herb for soothing skin inflammation, cuts, and wounds. It helps with healing and reducing scars.
   - How to Use: Apply calendula ointment or oil to irritated or inflamed skin.
   - Preparation: Use calendula-infused oil or ointment for topical application.
3. Tea Tree Oil (Melaleuca alternifolia)
   - Uses: Tea tree oil is widely used to treat acne, fungal infections, and minor skin irritations due to its antibacterial and antifungal properties.
   - How to Use: Apply diluted tea tree oil to acne-prone skin or fungal infections.
   - Preparation: Mix tea tree oil with a carrier oil (like coconut oil) before applying to the skin.
4. Chamomile (Matricaria chamomilla)
   - Uses: Chamomile is gentle on the skin and works well for treating conditions like eczema, dermatitis, and acne due to its anti-inflammatory properties.

How to Use: Apply chamomile tea as a compress or use chamomile-infused oil to soothe irritated skin.

- **Preparation**: Brew chamomile tea and use it as a compress or add chamomile essential oil to your skincare products.
5. **Witch Hazel (Hamamelis virginiana)**
    - **Uses**: Witch hazel is great for treating acne, skin irritation, and inflammation. It acts as an astringent and helps tighten and tone the skin.
    - **How to Use**: Apply witch hazel extract directly to the skin to help reduce acne and irritation.
    - **Preparation**: Use witch hazel extract as a toner after cleansing your face, or apply it with a cotton ball to affected areas.

Herbal remedies offer a natural and holistic approach to managing common ailments like colds, digestive issues, stress, and skin conditions. Many of these herbs are easy to incorporate into your daily routine, whether through teas, tinctures, oils, or topical applications. Always consult with a healthcare provider before starting any herbal remedy, especially if you are pregnant, nursing, or have pre-existing health conditions.

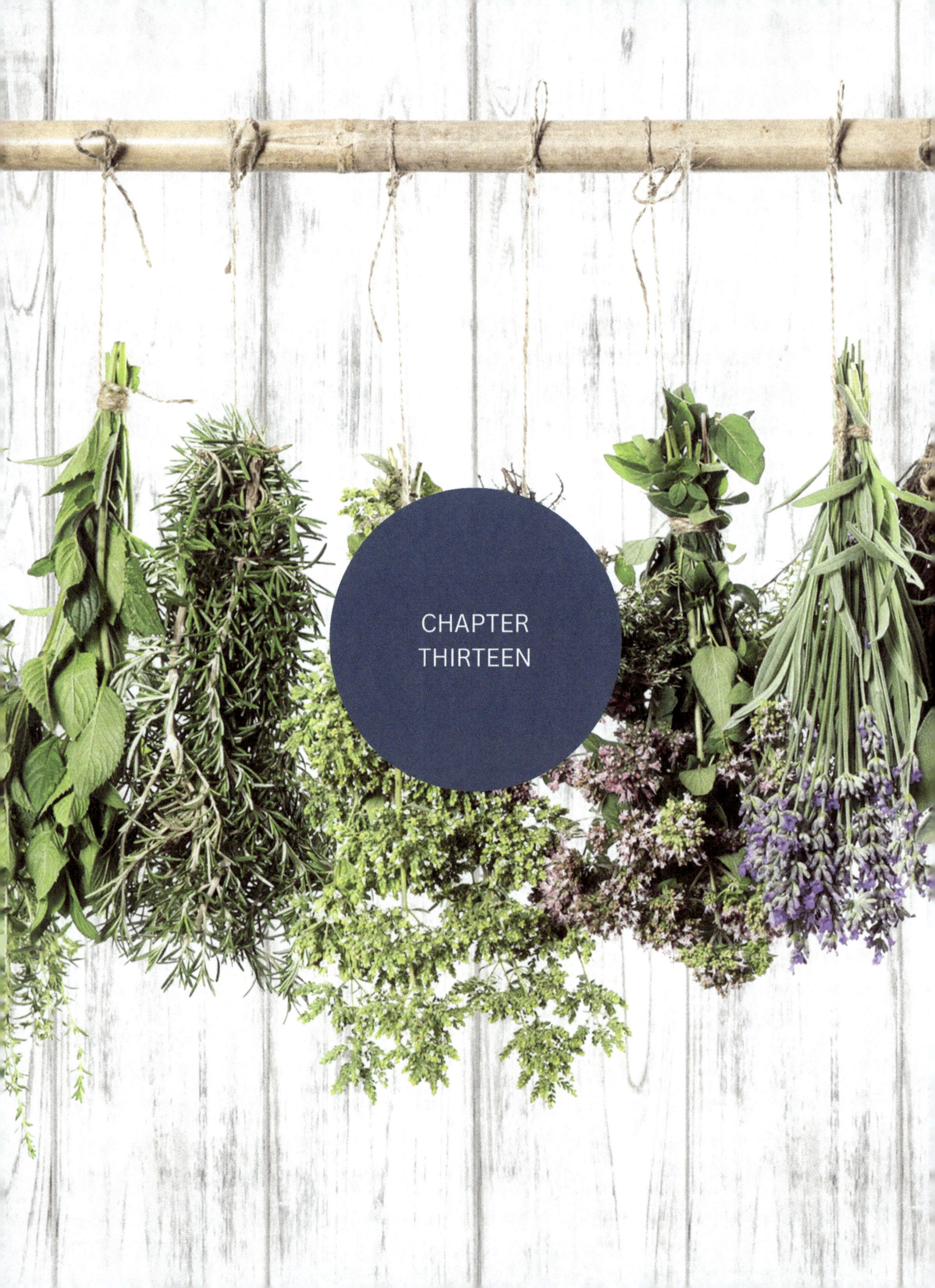

CHAPTER THIRTEEN

Herbal Support for Women's Health

Herbal remedies have long been used to support women's health at various stages of life, including menstrual health, fertility, and menopause. Herbs can provide natural relief from common issues such as menstrual cramps, hormonal imbalances, and menopause-related symptoms. Below are some of the most effective herbs for supporting women's health at different stages of life.

Menstrual Health

Menstrual issues such as cramps, heavy bleeding, and irregular cycles are common problems faced by many women. Several herbs are known to help alleviate these symptoms and promote menstrual health.

1. Dong Quai (Angelica sinensis)
   - Uses: Dong Quai is often referred to as the "female ginseng" and is commonly used in traditional Chinese medicine to regulate the menstrual cycle, relieve cramps, and balance hormones.
   - How to Use: Dong Quai can be taken as a tincture, tea, or in capsule form. It is often combined with other herbs to enhance its effects on menstrual health.
   - Preparation: Steep Dong Quai root in hot water to make a soothing tea. It can also be used in formulas for regulating menstruation.
2. Chaste Tree (Vitex agnus-castus)
   - Uses: Chaste tree, also known as Vitex, is one of the most popular herbs for regulating menstrual cycles and balancing hormones. It helps alleviate symptoms of PMS, including irritability, bloating, and breast tenderness.
   - How to Use: Take as a tincture, capsule, or tea. It is often used for a few months to see significant improvements in menstrual symptoms.
   - Preparation: Brew chaste tree leaves or berries in hot water to make a gentle tea, or take a tincture to balance hormones.

1. **Red Clover (Trifolium pratense)**
   - **Uses**: Red clover is high in phytoestrogens, which are plant-based compounds that mimic estrogen in the body. It is beneficial for balancing hormones, alleviating menstrual cramps, and improving overall menstrual health.
   - **How to Use**: Drink red clover tea, or take as a tincture or capsule to support reproductive health.
   - **Preparation**: Steep dried red clover flowers in boiling water for about 10 minutes to create a soothing tea.
2. **Cinnamon (Cinnamomum verum)**
   - **Uses**: Cinnamon is known for its ability to reduce menstrual cramps and regulate menstrual flow. It also helps with irregular periods and can ease bloating.
   - **How to Use**: Add cinnamon to your diet in teas, smoothies, or meals. Cinnamon is particularly effective when consumed at the start of the menstrual cycle.
   - **Preparation**: Brew cinnamon sticks in hot water, or sprinkle ground cinnamon in warm beverages like tea or smoothies.
3. **Ginger (Zingiber officinale)**
   - **Uses**: Ginger has anti-inflammatory properties that make it effective for relieving menstrual cramps, nausea, and other menstrual discomforts.
   - **How to Use**: Drink ginger tea or chew on fresh ginger slices. Ginger can also be taken in capsule form for quicker relief.
   - **Preparation**: Slice fresh ginger root and steep it in hot water for a soothing and anti-inflammatory tea.

Fertility Support

Many women use herbal remedies to support fertility and balance reproductive hormones. Herbs can help improve the overall health of the reproductive system and support the body in preparing for conception.

1. Raspberry Leaf (Rubus idaeus)
    - Uses: Raspberry leaf is known for its ability to tone the uterus, regulate menstrual cycles, and support fertility. It is especially helpful for women trying to conceive and those in the later stages of pregnancy.
    - How to Use: Raspberry leaf tea can be consumed regularly to help support a healthy reproductive system. It is often recommended during the pre-conception phase to enhance fertility.
    - Preparation: Steep dried raspberry leaves in boiling water for 10-15 minutes to create a nourishing tea.
2. Maca Root (Lepidium meyenii)
    - Uses: Maca root is an adaptogen that supports hormonal balance, increases energy, and improves libido. It is often used to enhance fertility in both men and women by regulating hormones and increasing fertility potential.
    - How to Use: Maca root is available in powder, capsule, or tincture form. It is commonly added to smoothies or shakes.
    - Preparation: Add maca powder to smoothies or mix with water or juice.
3. Tribulus Terrestris
    - Uses: Tribulus is commonly used to enhance fertility by improving ovulation and regulating menstrual cycles. It also helps improve libido and support overall reproductive health.
    - How to Use: Take as a capsule or in tincture form. Tribulus is best taken regularly for several months for maximum effect.
    - Preparation: Tribulus tinctures can be found in most herbal stores, and capsules can be taken according to the recommended dosage.

4. **Shatavari (Asparagus racemosus)**
    - **Uses**: Shatavari is a well-known herb in Ayurvedic medicine that supports female reproductive health. It enhances fertility by balancing hormones and improving the quality of eggs and uterine health.
    - **How to Use**: Shatavari is available in powder, capsule, or tincture form. It can be taken daily to support overall reproductive health.
    - **Preparation**: Mix Shatavari powder with warm water or milk, or take capsules as recommended.
5. **Dong Quai (Angelica sinensis)**
    - **Uses**: In addition to regulating menstruation, Dong Quai is also beneficial for fertility. It helps balance estrogen levels, improve blood flow to the uterus, and improve overall reproductive health.
    - **How to Use**: Take Dong Quai as a tincture, capsule, or tea to help balance hormones and promote fertility.
    - **Preparation**: Brew Dong Quai root in hot water to make a soothing tea or take a tincture before ovulation.

Menopause Support

Menopause is a natural transition in a woman's life, but it can come with challenging symptoms, including hot flashes, mood swings, night sweats, and vaginal dryness. Many herbs can help ease these symptoms and provide relief during this time of life.

1. Black Cohosh (Actaea racemosa)
    - Uses: Black Cohosh is one of the most widely used herbs for managing menopause symptoms, particularly hot flashes, mood swings, and night sweats.
    - How to Use: Take Black Cohosh in capsule, tablet, or tincture form. It is often used in combination with other herbs to manage menopausal symptoms.
    - Preparation: Black Cohosh can be taken as a tincture or in capsule form. It is most effective when used regularly.
2. Red Clover (Trifolium pratense)
    - Uses: Red clover contains phytoestrogens, which mimic estrogen in the body. It helps manage menopausal symptoms like hot flashes, night sweats, and vaginal dryness.
    - How to Use: Drink red clover tea or take in capsule or tincture form to ease menopausal symptoms.
    - Preparation: Brew red clover flowers in hot water for a calming tea that may help alleviate hot flashes and other symptoms.
3. Soy Isoflavones
    - Uses: Soy isoflavones are plant compounds that act as phytoestrogens, which can help balance estrogen levels in the body and relieve symptoms of menopause, including hot flashes and night sweats.
    - How to Use: Incorporate soy-based foods like tofu, tempeh, and soy milk into your diet, or take soy isoflavones in supplement form.
    - Preparation: Consume soy products in your daily meals or take soy isoflavone supplements as directed.

4. **Sage (Salvia officinalis)**
    - **Uses**: Sage has traditionally been used to reduce hot flashes and night sweats associated with menopause. It can also help balance mood and reduce anxiety.
    - **How to Use**: Drink sage tea or use sage essential oil for aromatherapy to support hormonal balance during menopause.
    - **Preparation**: Steep fresh or dried sage leaves in hot water for a cooling, calming tea.
5. **Maca Root (Lepidium meyenii)**
    - **Uses**: Maca root helps balance hormones and improve energy levels during menopause. It is also beneficial for reducing mood swings and hot flashes.
    - **How to Use**: Maca root powder can be added to smoothies or taken as capsules to support overall hormone balance during menopause.
    - **Preparation**: Blend maca root powder into smoothies, or take capsules regularly.

Herbal remedies offer valuable support to women throughout all stages of life. Whether you're looking to regulate your menstrual cycle, support fertility, or ease the symptoms of menopause, there are many herbs that can help. Always consult with a healthcare provider before starting any new herbal regimen, especially if you're pregnant, nursing, or on other medications. Herbs can be a powerful ally in promoting women's health naturally and effectively.

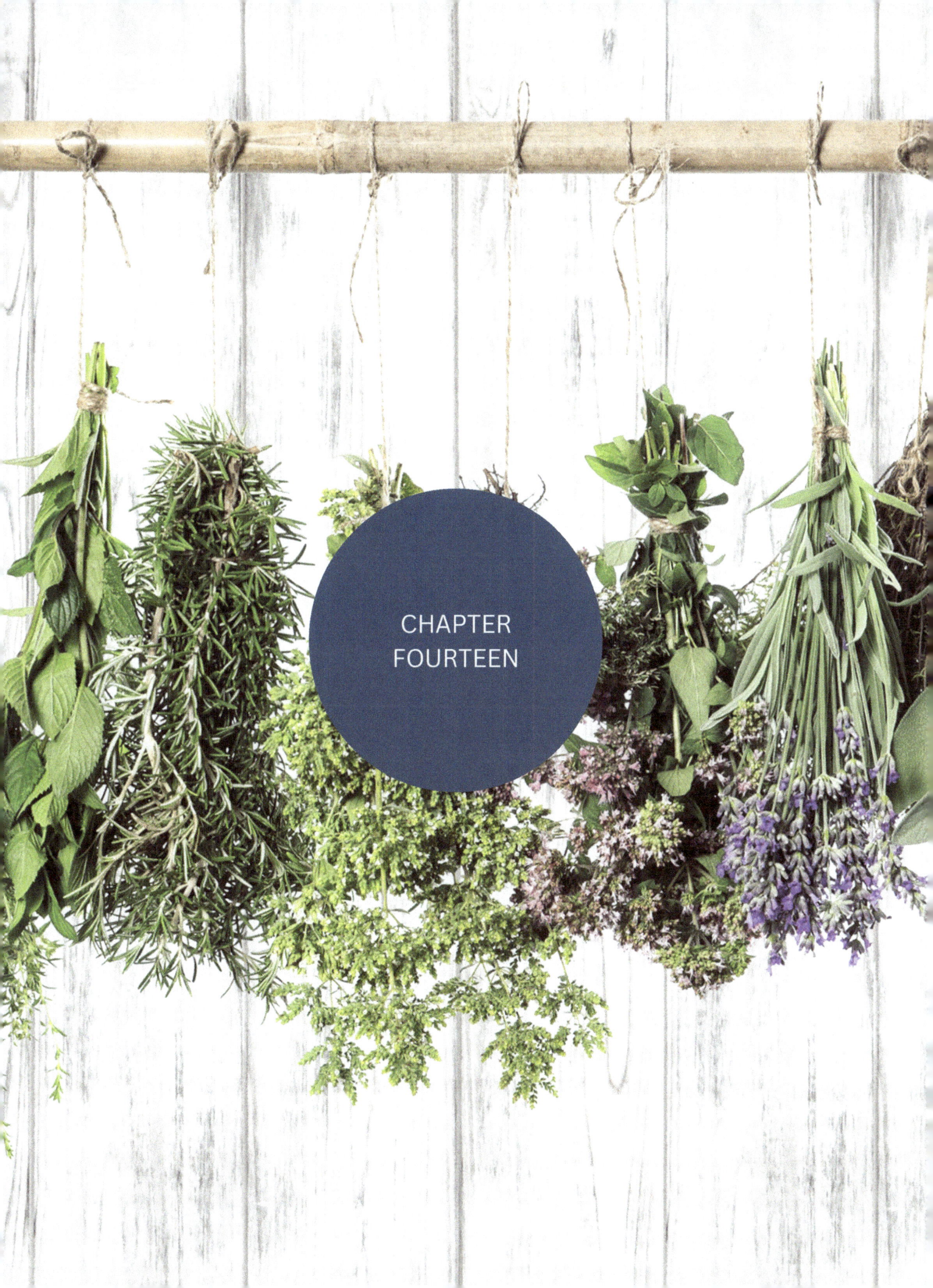

CHAPTER FOURTEEN

Herbs for Men's Wellness

Men's wellness encompasses a range of health concerns, including energy, stamina, prostate health, and sexual vitality. Herbal remedies have long been used to support men's health, offering natural solutions to common issues such as low energy, stress, erectile dysfunction, and prostate problems. Below are some of the most beneficial herbs that support men's overall health and vitality.

Energy and Stamina

Men, especially those with active lifestyles or demanding schedules, often seek natural remedies to boost energy levels, endurance, and physical stamina. Herbal support can help combat fatigue and increase vitality.

1. Ginseng (Panax ginseng)
   - Uses: Ginseng is a powerful adaptogen that has been used for centuries to improve energy, stamina, and overall vitality. It helps reduce fatigue, boosts physical endurance, and enhances mental clarity. Ginseng is also known for improving sexual performance and supporting hormonal balance.
   - How to Use: Ginseng is available in tincture, capsule, or tea form. It can be taken daily to support energy levels, especially during periods of stress or fatigue.
   - Preparation: Brew ginseng root in hot water to make an invigorating tea, or take a capsule or tincture for more concentrated effects.
2. Maca Root (Lepidium meyenii)

Uses: Maca is an adaptogenic herb that is widely used to enhance energy levels, endurance, and stamina. It supports adrenal function, improves mood, and promotes a healthy libido. Maca is also known for its ability to balance hormones and combat fatigue.

- **How to Use**: Maca is typically consumed in powder form, which can be added to smoothies, juices, or protein shakes. It is also available in capsule or tincture form.
- **Preparation**: Add maca root powder to smoothies or drinks, or take it in capsule form for enhanced stamina.

3. **Rhodiola (Rhodiola rosea)**
    - **Uses**: Rhodiola is an adaptogen that helps the body manage stress and fatigue. It is commonly used to increase energy, improve stamina, and enhance mental performance. Rhodiola has also been shown to help boost libido and reduce symptoms of depression and anxiety.
    - **How to Use**: Rhodiola is available as a tincture, capsule, or powder. It can be taken daily to promote energy, mental clarity, and physical endurance.
    - **Preparation**: Rhodiola powder can be mixed into smoothies, or the tincture can be taken in small doses for quick effects.
4. **Ashwagandha (Withania somnifera)**
    - **Uses**: Ashwagandha is a powerful adaptogen that helps the body cope with stress while boosting energy levels and stamina. It promotes endurance, muscle strength, and recovery after physical activity. Ashwagandha also supports male fertility and enhances overall vitality.
    - **How to Use**: Ashwagandha is available in capsule, powder, or tincture form. It can be taken daily to improve stamina and energy levels.
    - **Preparation**: Mix ashwagandha powder into milk or smoothies, or take it in capsule form for a boost in energy and stamina.

5. **Cordyceps (Cordyceps sinensis)**
    - **Uses**: Cordyceps is a medicinal mushroom known for its ability to enhance physical performance and stamina. It improves oxygen uptake, endurance, and energy production. It is often used by athletes and those seeking to improve their physical fitness.
    - **How to Use**: Cordyceps is available in powder, capsule, or tincture form. It can be taken daily to boost energy levels and endurance.
    - **Preparation**: Add cordyceps powder to smoothies, or take it in capsule form to increase energy and stamina.

Prostate Health

Prostate health is an important concern for men, particularly as they age. Herbal remedies can support prostate function, reduce symptoms of benign prostatic hyperplasia (BPH), and maintain overall urinary and reproductive health.

1. Saw Palmetto (Serenoa repens)
    - Uses: Saw palmetto is one of the most widely used herbs for supporting prostate health. It is especially effective for managing symptoms of BPH, such as frequent urination and reduced urinary flow. Saw palmetto works by inhibiting the enzyme responsible for converting testosterone into dihydrotestosterone (DHT), a hormone linked to prostate enlargement.
    - How to Use: Saw palmetto is available in capsules, tablets, or tincture form. It is commonly taken daily to maintain prostate health and alleviate urinary symptoms associated with BPH.
    - Preparation: Saw palmetto capsules are often taken in the recommended dose, or the tincture can be used as directed.
2. Nettle Root (Urtica dioica)
    - Uses: Nettle root is known for its ability to support prostate health by promoting healthy urine flow and reducing the symptoms of BPH. It contains compounds that help inhibit the growth of prostate cells and maintain normal urinary function.
    - How to Use: Nettle root is available in capsule or tincture form. It is often used in combination with saw palmetto to provide comprehensive support for prostate health.
    - Preparation: Take nettle root in capsule form or use the tincture as directed to support prostate function.

3. **Pumpkin Seed (Cucurbita pepo)**
    - **Uses**: Pumpkin seeds are rich in zinc, which is essential for prostate health. They have anti-inflammatory properties and can help reduce symptoms of BPH, such as frequent urination and nighttime urination. Pumpkin seed oil is often used to support urinary and prostate health.
    - **How to Use**: Pumpkin seeds can be eaten raw, roasted, or taken as pumpkin seed oil in capsule form. The oil is often used to promote healthy prostate function.
    - **Preparation**: Snack on raw pumpkin seeds, add them to salads or smoothies, or take pumpkin seed oil in capsule form.
4. **Pygeum (Prunus africana)**
    - **Uses**: Pygeum is a tree native to Africa, and its bark has been traditionally used to treat symptoms of BPH. It helps reduce inflammation in the prostate and urinary tract, improving urine flow and decreasing the frequency of nighttime urination.
    - **How to Use**: Pygeum is typically available in capsule or tablet form. It can be taken daily to support prostate health and reduce symptoms of BPH.
    - **Preparation**: Take pygeum in capsule form or as a tincture to support prostate health.
5. **Tomato (Lycopersicon esculentum)**
    - **Uses**: Tomatoes are rich in lycopene, a powerful antioxidant that has been shown to help maintain prostate health and reduce the risk of prostate cancer. Lycopene helps reduce oxidative stress and inflammation in the prostate.
    - **How to Use**: Eating fresh tomatoes or drinking tomato juice is an easy way to incorporate this beneficial compound into your diet. Tomato paste and cooked tomatoes are also great sources of lycopene.
    - **Preparation**: Incorporate tomatoes into your diet through salads, soups, or sauces, or drink fresh tomato juice to support prostate health.

Sexual Health and Libido

Herbal support for men's sexual health is widely sought after, with many herbs known for their ability to enhance libido, improve sexual performance, and support healthy testosterone levels.

1. Tribulus Terrestris
   - Uses: Tribulus is commonly used to enhance libido and sexual function by increasing testosterone levels. It is known to improve erectile function and support overall male vitality.
   - How to Use: Tribulus is typically taken as a supplement in capsule or tincture form. It can be taken regularly to enhance sexual performance and energy levels.
   - Preparation: Take tribulus in capsule or tincture form as directed to boost libido and sexual health.
2. Horny Goat Weed (Epimedium)
   - Uses: Horny goat weed is an herb traditionally used to treat erectile dysfunction and boost sexual desire. It contains icariin, which helps increase blood flow to the genital area, promoting stronger erections and improving libido.
   - How to Use: Horny goat weed is commonly available in capsule or tincture form. It can be taken regularly to enhance sexual performance.
   - Preparation: Take horny goat weed as a supplement in the recommended dose to boost libido and sexual vitality.
3. Gingko Biloba (Ginkgo biloba)
   - Uses: Ginkgo biloba is known for improving circulation, which can be especially beneficial for men with erectile dysfunction. It increases blood flow to the genitals and helps improve sexual function.
   - How to Use: Ginkgo biloba is typically taken as a supplement or in tea form. It is often used for improving circulation and enhancing sexual performance.
   - Preparation: Take ginkgo biloba capsules or drink ginkgo tea to support sexual health.

Herbal remedies provide valuable support for men's wellness, particularly for energy, stamina, and prostate health. Whether you're looking to enhance vitality, improve sexual function, or maintain prostate health, these herbs offer natural and effective solutions. Always consult with a healthcare provider before starting any new herbal regimen, especially if you have pre-existing health conditions or are taking other medications. Herbs can be a powerful ally in supporting men's health and vitality throughout life.

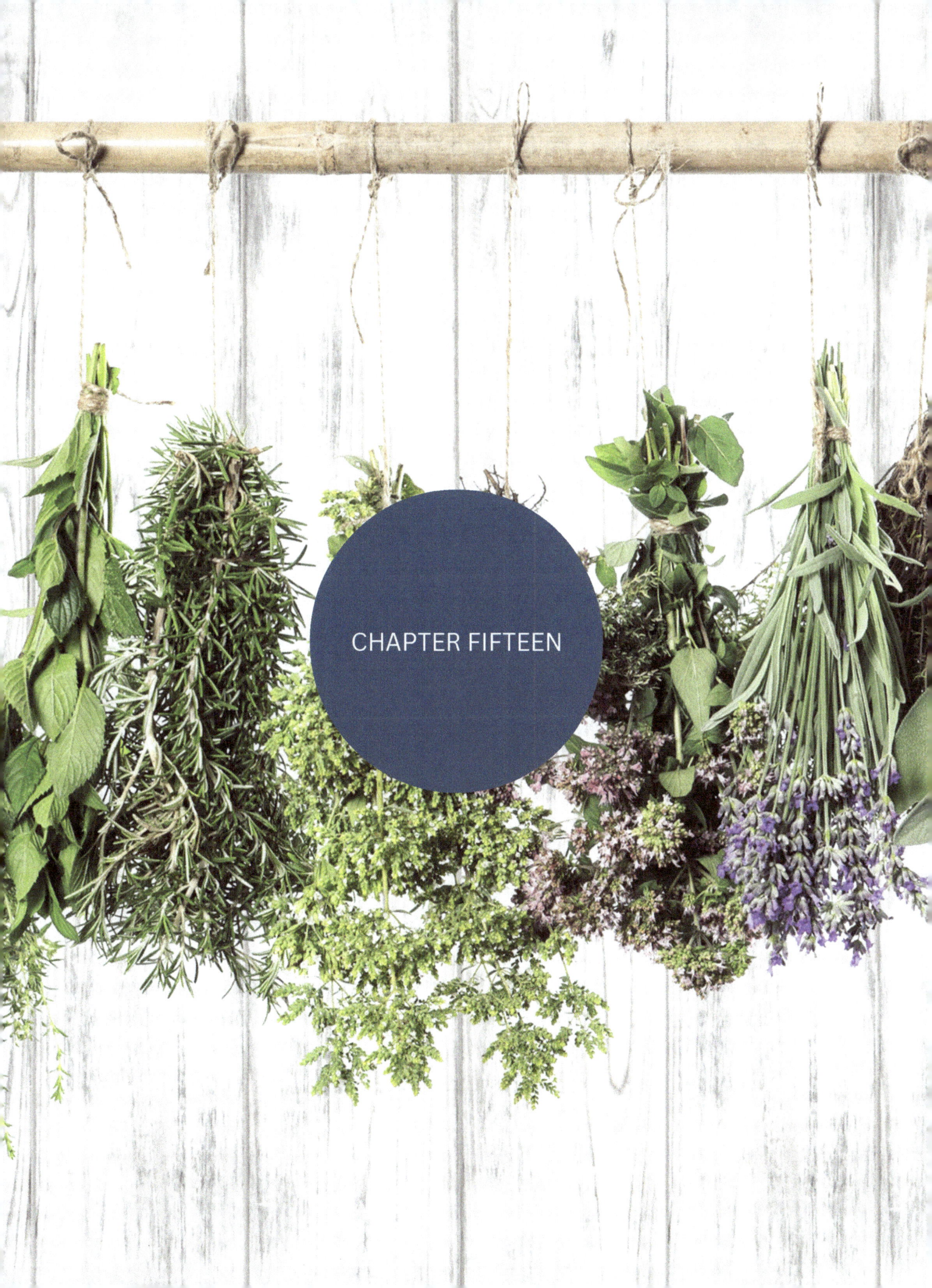

CHAPTER FIFTEEN

Herbs for Children

Herbs can be powerful allies in promoting health and healing for children, providing gentle, natural remedies for common childhood ailments. These herbs are typically milder and safer for children when used appropriately, making them an excellent alternative to pharmaceuticals for minor health concerns. Below are some herbs commonly used for children's health and wellness.

Gentle Remedies for Childhood Illnesses
1. Chamomile (Matricaria chamomilla)
    - Uses: Chamomile is well known for its calming effects, making it an excellent herb for children who have trouble sleeping, are feeling anxious, or suffer from digestive issues. It can soothe upset stomachs, alleviate colic in infants, and help with mild irritability and restlessness.
    - How to Use: Chamomile can be given as a tea, infused in a warm bath, or used as a tincture. It's safe for children and can help ease minor digestive discomforts, such as bloating or constipation.
    - Preparation: Brew chamomile tea for children, ensuring it's mild and not too concentrated. For infants, a diluted chamomile tea can help soothe colic.
2. Lemon Balm (Melissa officinalis)
    - Uses: Lemon balm is another calming herb that promotes relaxation and can help relieve symptoms of mild anxiety, stress, and insomnia. It is also used to ease digestive issues such as indigestion and gas.
    - How to Use: Lemon balm is often used as a tea or tincture. It is particularly helpful for children who are nervous, irritable, or experiencing sleep difficulties.
    - Preparation: Brew a mild lemon balm tea for children or add a few drops of tincture (diluted) to their water to calm nerves and promote a restful night's sleep.

3. **Echinacea (Echinacea purpurea)**
    - **Uses**: Echinacea is widely known for its immune-boosting properties and is commonly used to prevent or reduce the severity of colds and flu. It helps stimulate the immune system, making it a great option for children during cold and flu season.
    - **How to Use**: Echinacea can be given as a tincture, in capsule form (for older children), or as an herbal tea. It's generally safe for children over the age of 2.
    - **Preparation**: Echinacea tea or tincture can be given to children in small, diluted doses to help fight off colds and infections. Always consult a healthcare provider before giving echinacea to children with allergies to ragweed.
4. **Ginger (Zingiber officinale)**
    - **Uses**: Ginger is a great remedy for nausea, motion sickness, and digestive discomfort. It helps stimulate the digestive system and can soothe upset stomachs, making it particularly useful for children who suffer from nausea or digestive upset.
    - **How to Use**: Ginger can be used in a mild tea or as a dried powder added to food. It can also be taken in capsule form, though children may prefer it as a tea or even in syrup form for younger children.
    - **Preparation**: Brew a mild ginger tea, or mix a pinch of ginger powder into food or smoothies for children who suffer from nausea or indigestion.
5. **Peppermint (Mentha piperita)**
    - **Uses**: Peppermint is a wonderful herb for relieving digestive discomfort, such as bloating, indigestion, and gas. It is also used for soothing headaches and colicky babies, making it a versatile remedy for children.
    - **How to Use**: Peppermint is usually given as tea or as a diluted tincture. It's important to use peppermint in moderation, as it can be too strong for very young children

Preparation: Make a mild peppermint tea for children with digestive discomfort. For babies, you can apply diluted peppermint oil (on the soles of their feet) or add a few drops to their bath to help ease colic.

6. **Marshmallow Root (Althaea officinalis)**
    - **Uses**: Marshmallow root is a gentle herb known for its soothing properties, particularly for sore throats, coughs, and gastrointestinal issues. It helps reduce inflammation and coat the mucous membranes, providing relief from dry coughs and irritated throats.
    - **How to Use**: Marshmallow root can be used in teas, syrups, or tinctures. It's safe for children and particularly helpful when a cough or sore throat is present.
    - **Preparation**: Brew marshmallow root as an herbal tea to soothe a child's sore throat or cough. You can also make marshmallow root syrup to coat the throat and relieve irritation.

7. **Slippery Elm (Ulmus rubra)**
    - **Uses**: Slippery elm is similar to marshmallow root in that it is known for its ability to soothe irritated mucous membranes, especially in the digestive tract. It helps with conditions like diarrhea, constipation, and sore throats.
    - **How to Use**: Slippery elm is commonly used as a powder mixed with water to create a soothing drink or paste. It can be taken as tea or in capsule form.
    - **Preparation**: Mix slippery elm powder into a smooth drink or give it as a tea to children suffering from digestive discomfort or a sore throat.

8. **Fennel (Foeniculum vulgare)**
    - **Uses**: Fennel is great for digestive issues in children, particularly colic, gas, and bloating. It can also help relieve mild constipation. Fennel's natural antispasmodic properties make it useful for easing stomach cramps.

How to Use: Fennel seeds can be brewed into a tea, or fennel oil can be applied topically in a diluted form to ease abdominal discomfort.

- **Preparation**: Brew fennel tea for infants and toddlers to help alleviate gas and colic, or give older children a mild fennel tea for digestive support.

9. **Licorice Root (Glycyrrhiza glabra)**
    - **Uses**: Licorice root is known for its ability to soothe sore throats, reduce coughing, and relieve digestive issues. It is often used for respiratory health and can help support children with coughs or colds.
    - **How to Use**: Licorice root can be used in teas, lozenges, or syrups. However, it should be used sparingly in children due to its potency.
    - **Preparation**: Prepare a mild licorice tea or syrup for children who are suffering from a cough or sore throat. Use in moderation, and avoid for children with high blood pressure.

10. **Lavender (Lavandula angustifolia)**
    - **Uses**: Lavender is well known for its calming properties. It is useful for children with anxiety, stress, or difficulty sleeping. Lavender can also relieve headaches and ease upset stomachs.
    - **How to Use**: Lavender is often used in aromatherapy, in teas, or in a soothing bath. It can also be applied topically (diluted) to help with skin irritation or anxiety.
    - **Preparation**: Use lavender essential oil in a diffuser to calm children before bedtime, or prepare a mild lavender tea for soothing digestive discomfort or anxiety.

Safety Considerations for Herbs for Children

While herbs can be gentle and effective for children, it's important to always use them cautiously. Some herbs, even though natural, may not be suitable for very young children or infants. Here are a few tips to ensure the safety of herbal remedies for children:

- Consult a pediatrician before introducing any herbs, especially if your child has underlying health conditions or is taking medications.
- Use age-appropriate doses: Always adjust doses for age and weight, and use mild concentrations of herbs.
- Monitor for allergies: Introduce new herbs one at a time and monitor for any allergic reactions.
- Avoid certain herbs: Some herbs, such as pennyroyal and comfrey, are not recommended for children due to their potency or toxicity in large doses.

Herbs can be a safe and gentle way to address common childhood health issues, from digestive discomfort and colds to stress and sleep difficulties. By choosing appropriate herbs and using them in the correct doses, you can offer your child the natural healing power of plants. As with any natural remedy, always seek guidance from a healthcare provider to ensure the safety and suitability of herbs for your child's specific needs.

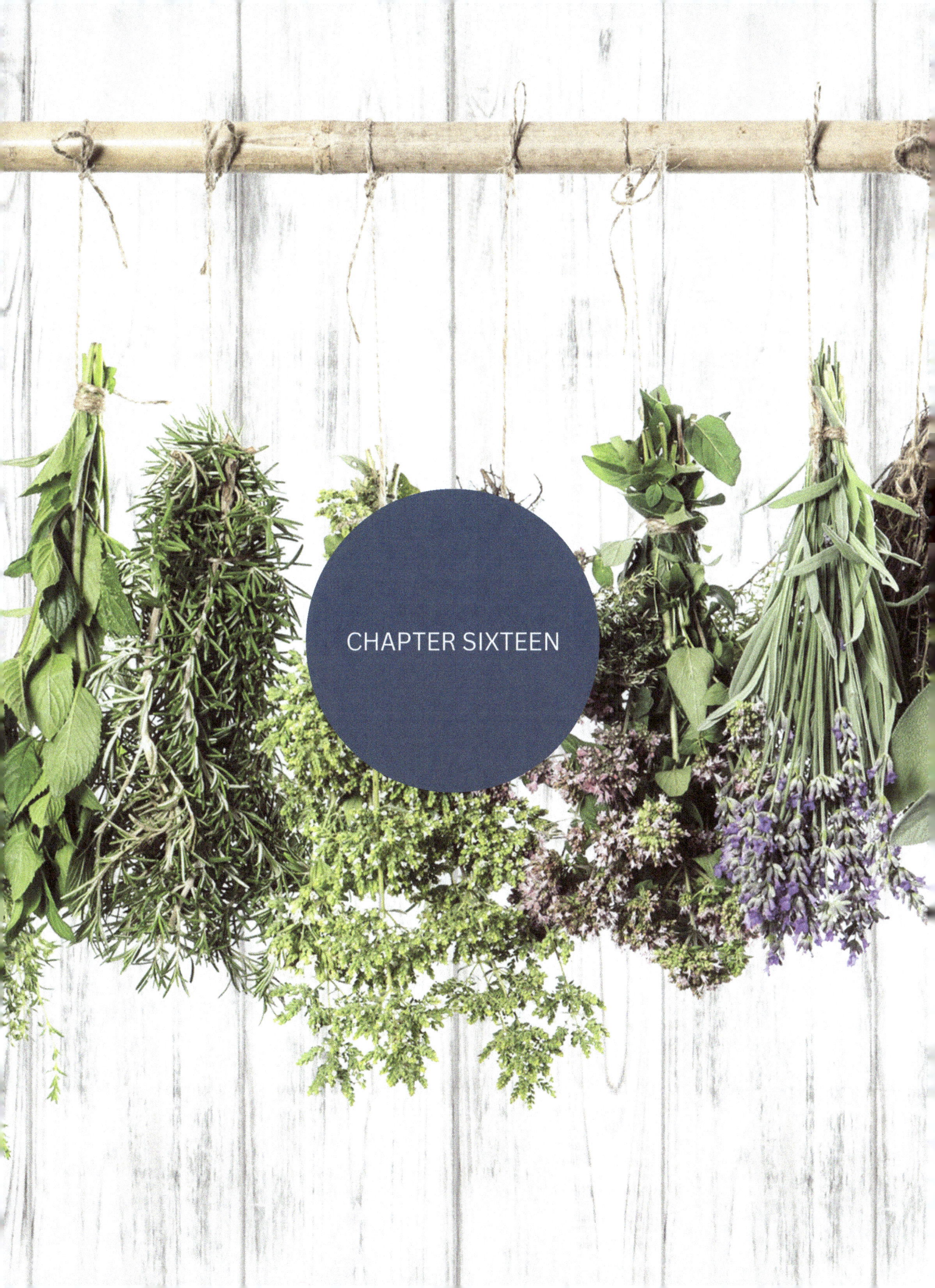

CHAPTER SIXTEEN

Eldercare with Herbs: Cognitive Support and Chronic Pain Relief

Herbs have long been used to support the health and well-being of older adults, offering natural solutions for many of the common challenges faced as we age. Among the most critical concerns for the elderly are cognitive decline and chronic pain. Many herbs have been identified as beneficial in addressing these issues, either by improving cognitive function or providing relief from pain. Below is a detailed exploration of key herbs that can support cognitive health and alleviate chronic pain in elderly individuals.

Cognitive Support for the Elderly

As individuals age, cognitive function may begin to decline, leading to issues such as memory loss, mental confusion, and difficulty with concentration. These challenges are often associated with conditions like dementia and Alzheimer's disease. Fortunately, several herbs are known to support brain health and enhance cognitive performance. Here are some of the most promising herbs for cognitive support in elderly care:

1. Ginkgo Biloba (Ginkgo biloba)
    - Uses: Ginkgo biloba is one of the most widely studied herbs for cognitive health. It has been shown to improve memory, focus, and overall mental clarity, especially in individuals with age-related cognitive decline. Ginkgo is believed to increase blood flow to the brain, supporting the health of brain cells and improving cognitive function.
    - How to Use: Ginkgo can be taken in tablet, capsule, or liquid extract form. It is often recommended for individuals experiencing early stages of cognitive decline or those seeking to boost memory and concentration.
    - Preparation: A standardized extract is typically the most effective form, with doses ranging from 120 to 240 mg per day, divided into two or three doses.

1. **Bacopa (Bacopa monnieri)**
   - **Uses**: Bacopa, also known as Brahmi, is an herb used in Ayurvedic medicine to enhance memory and cognitive function. Studies have shown that Bacopa can improve cognitive performance, enhance memory retention, and reduce anxiety. It is believed to work by supporting the production of certain neurotransmitters associated with learning and memory.
   - **How to Use**: Bacopa can be consumed in powdered form, capsules, or as a tincture. It is most effective when taken consistently over a period of time, as its cognitive-enhancing effects tend to build gradually.
   - **Preparation**: Typically, 300 mg of Bacopa extract, standardized to 50% bacosides, is taken daily to support mental clarity and memory.
2. **Rosemary (Rosmarinus officinalis)**
   - **Uses**: Rosemary has long been considered a herb for mental clarity and cognitive function. It is thought to stimulate circulation, particularly in the brain, and can help improve memory and focus. It also has antioxidant properties that protect the brain from age-related damage.
   - **How to Use**: Rosemary can be used as a tea, taken as a tincture, or even inhaled as an essential oil. Drinking rosemary tea or using the oil in aromatherapy may help improve focus and cognitive function.

Preparation: A cup of rosemary tea can be made by steeping a few sprigs of fresh rosemary or a teaspoon of dried rosemary in hot water for 5-10 minutes. It can be consumed once or twice a day.

3. Ashwagandha (Withania somnifera)
    - Uses: Ashwagandha, an adaptogenic herb from Ayurvedic tradition, is known to help reduce stress and anxiety, which can significantly affect cognitive performance in older adults. It can also improve memory and promote overall mental well-being by balancing cortisol levels, a hormone linked to stress.
    - How to Use: Ashwagandha can be taken in capsule form or as a powder mixed with warm milk or water. It is especially beneficial for those who experience mental fatigue or stress-related cognitive decline.
    - Preparation: A common dose is 300–500 mg of standardized extract per day, but it's best to consult a healthcare professional for personalized advice.

4, **Turmeric (Curcuma longa)**
- **Uses**: Turmeric contains curcumin, a compound with potent anti-inflammatory and antioxidant properties. It has been shown to improve cognitive function and may help prevent or slow the progression of conditions like Alzheimer's disease. Curcumin is thought to reduce inflammation in the brain and increase the production of neuroprotective proteins.
- **How to Use**: Turmeric can be consumed in food, as a tea, or in supplement form. Combining turmeric with black pepper, which contains piperine, enhances curcumin absorption.

Preparation: Turmeric tea can be made by boiling fresh or dried turmeric root with water, or it can be taken in capsule form, typically in doses of 500–1,000 mg per day.

Chronic Pain Relief for the Elderly

Chronic pain, including conditions like arthritis, back pain, and neuropathy, is common in older adults. Many herbs have been traditionally used to provide natural pain relief, reduce inflammation, and support joint health. Here are some of the best herbs for managing chronic pain in elderly individuals:

1. Devil's Claw (Harpagophytum procumbens)
    - Uses: Devil's claw is commonly used to relieve pain associated with osteoarthritis, back pain, and other inflammatory conditions. It has natural anti-inflammatory and analgesic properties, making it effective for reducing joint pain and improving mobility.
    - How to Use: Devil's claw is typically taken as a standardized extract in tablet or capsule form. It may also be used in topical creams for localized pain relief.
    - Preparation: A common dose is 600–1,200 mg of standardized extract daily. It should be used with caution in individuals with heart conditions or those on blood pressure medication.
2. Willow Bark (Salix alba)
    - Uses: Willow bark contains salicin, a compound similar to aspirin, and has been used for centuries to relieve pain and reduce inflammation. It is particularly effective for conditions like arthritis, back pain, and headaches.
    - How to Use: Willow bark can be taken as a tea, in capsule form, or as a tincture. It should be used with care in individuals who are sensitive to aspirin or who are on blood-thinning medications.
    - Preparation: Willow bark tea can be made by steeping 1-2 teaspoons of dried bark in hot water for 10 minutes. Alternatively, capsules containing 60–120 mg of standardized extract can be taken daily.

3. **Turmeric (Curcuma longa)**
    - **Uses**: In addition to its cognitive benefits, turmeric's anti-inflammatory properties make it an effective remedy for chronic pain, especially in conditions like arthritis. It helps reduce joint swelling and improves mobility.
    - **How to Use**: Turmeric can be consumed as a supplement, added to food, or taken in tea form. It works best when combined with black pepper, which enhances its bioavailability.
    - **Preparation**: A dose of 500–1,000 mg of turmeric extract, standardized to contain 95% curcumin, is typically recommended for pain relief.
4. **Ginger (Zingiber officinale)**
    - **Uses**: Ginger has natural anti-inflammatory and analgesic effects that can help alleviate pain caused by arthritis, muscle stiffness, and other chronic conditions. It can also reduce nausea, which may be helpful for elderly individuals dealing with pain medications.
    - **How to Use**: Ginger can be consumed as a tea, in capsule form, or added to meals. It can also be applied topically as a ginger-infused oil for pain relief.

Preparation: Ginger tea can be made by steeping fresh ginger slices in boiling water for 10 minutes. Alternatively, ginger supplements (1–2 grams per day) can be taken for chronic pain relief.

5. Capsaicin (Capsicum annuum)
    - Uses: Capsaicin, derived from chili peppers, is commonly used in topical creams and ointments to relieve localized pain, particularly from conditions like arthritis and neuropathy. It works by desensitizing pain receptors and reducing inflammation in the affected area.
    - How to Use: Capsaicin is most commonly used in creams and ointments. It should be applied to the painful area, with caution, to avoid skin irritation.
    - Preparation: Capsaicin creams are available over-the-counter and should be used as directed. They typically provide relief after consistent use over several days.

Herbs provide a natural and effective way to manage cognitive decline and chronic pain in elderly individuals. From supporting brain health with herbs like Ginkgo biloba and Bacopa to easing arthritis pain with Devil's claw and turmeric, the healing properties of plants offer many benefits for aging bodies. Always consult with a healthcare provider before introducing new herbs into an elderly person's routine, particularly if they are on medication or have pre-existing conditions. When used appropriately, herbs can play an integral role in enhancing the quality of life for older adults.

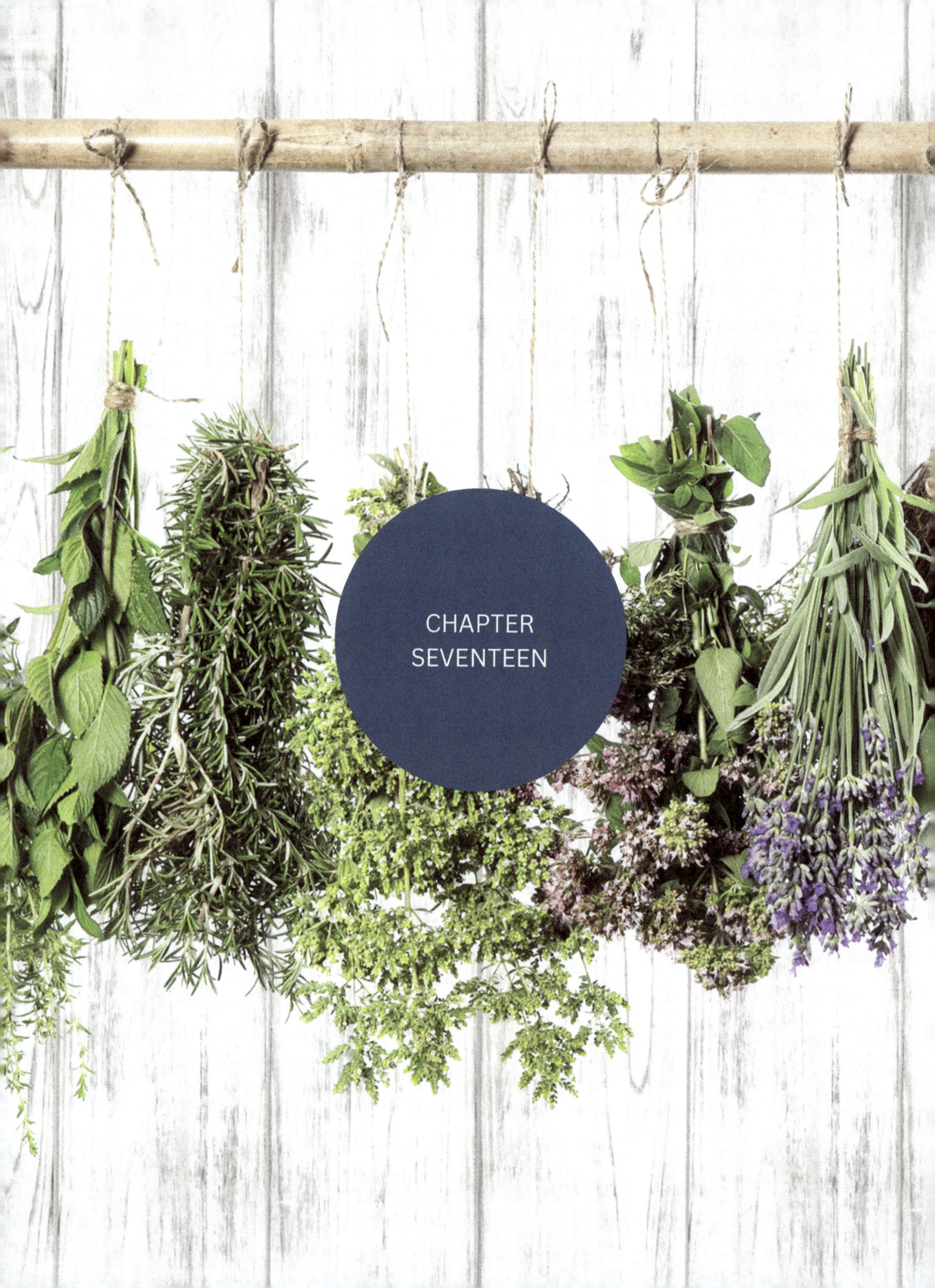

CHAPTER SEVENTEEN

The African Apothecary

Foraging and Growing African Herbs

Africa's rich biodiversity and deep-rooted traditional knowledge make it a continent rich in herbal healing practices. The African apothecary, steeped in centuries-old wisdom, draws on a vast array of herbs used for everything from treating common ailments to promoting overall well-being. Foraging and cultivating these plants have long been central to African cultures, and modern herbalists continue to draw on this indigenous knowledge to heal and nourish.

This chapter will explore the importance of foraging and growing African herbs, highlighting the most significant plants in African herbal medicine and offering practical advice for their cultivation. Whether for personal use or as part of a larger effort to preserve and protect African herbal heritage, the practice of gathering and growing herbs has much to offer.

The Importance of Foraging and Growing African Herbs

Foraging and growing herbs allow individuals to engage directly with nature, cultivating a relationship with plants that can offer numerous health benefits. Many African herbs have adapted to the continent's diverse climates, ranging from arid deserts to tropical rainforests. Their uses have been passed down from generation to generation, forming a cornerstone of African medicine.

Foraging allows individuals to access the fresh, potent properties of wild herbs, while growing herbs in a controlled environment can make these natural remedies more accessible, sustainable, and easier to use. Furthermore, cultivation ensures that these plants can be protected and preserved, contributing to biodiversity conservation efforts in the face of urbanization, climate change, and overharvesting.

Popular African Herbs and Their Uses

1. Moringa (Moringa oleifera)
    - Uses: Moringa, also known as the "drumstick tree," is known for its nutrient-rich leaves, which are used to treat malnutrition, boost energy, improve immune function, and manage blood sugar levels. Moringa's seeds are also used to purify water, and its oil has cosmetic uses.
    - Growing: Moringa is native to North Africa, though it has been spread across the continent and other tropical regions. It thrives in well-drained, sandy soil with plenty of sunlight. Growing moringa is relatively easy, requiring minimal water once established.
    - Foraging: Moringa grows naturally in many African regions, particularly in dry or semi-arid climates. When foraging, care should be taken to avoid harvesting from polluted areas, as moringa leaves and seeds are potent detoxifiers and should be free of contaminants.
2. Baobab (Adansonia digitata)
    - Uses: The baobab tree is iconic in Africa, with its fruit, seeds, and leaves being used for a variety of purposes. The fruit pulp is rich in vitamin C, antioxidants, and dietary fiber, while the seeds are used for medicinal oils and extracts. Baobab is known to improve immune health, combat inflammation, and support skin health.
    - Growing: Baobab trees can be found throughout Africa, particularly in the savannah and semi-arid regions. They prefer well-drained, sandy soils and are drought-tolerant, making them ideal for cultivation in dry regions. Baobab trees can be slow to mature, but they are long-lived and hardy.
    - Foraging: In the wild, baobab trees can be found across the African continent, with particularly large specimens in regions like West Africa. Harvesting the fruit involves collecting the pods, which can be opened to reveal the soft, tangy pulp inside.

1. **Devil's Claw (Harpagophytum procumbens)**
   - **Uses**: Known for its powerful anti-inflammatory and analgesic properties, Devil's claw is commonly used to treat joint pain, arthritis, and muscle soreness. It is also used for digestive issues and has mild laxative effects.
   - **Growing**: Native to southern Africa, Devil's claw thrives in arid and semi-arid climates. It is a low-growing, drought-tolerant plant that prefers sandy, well-drained soils. Cultivating Devil's claw requires patience, as it is a slow-growing plant that can take several years to mature.
   - **Foraging**: Devil's claw is often foraged from the wild in southern Africa, particularly in Namibia, Botswana, and South Africa. The tubers are the most commonly used part of the plant and are harvested after flowering.
2. **Hibiscus (Hibiscus sabdariffa)**
   - **Uses**: Hibiscus is widely used across Africa to prepare refreshing herbal teas, which are known for their ability to regulate blood pressure, support digestion, and provide antioxidants. Hibiscus flowers are also used in cosmetics and to treat inflammatory skin conditions.
   - **Growing**: Hibiscus thrives in tropical and subtropical climates, making it a common herb in many parts of Africa. It requires rich, well-drained soil and plenty of sunlight. Hibiscus plants can be grown in pots, making them suitable for urban environments.
   - **Foraging**: Hibiscus grows naturally in many regions of Africa, especially in hot, humid areas. The flowers are harvested when they are fully bloomed to be dried and used in teas, tinctures, and extracts.
3. **Neem (Azadirachta indica)**
   - **Uses**: Often referred to as the "village pharmacy," neem has extensive uses in traditional African medicine, from treating skin conditions to promoting oral health. It is also used to treat malaria, fevers, and infections due to its antimicrobial, antifungal, and antiviral properties.

- **Growing**: Neem is native to tropical and subtropical regions of Africa, particularly in the savannah. It grows best in well-drained soils with moderate water needs. Neem trees are drought-tolerant and can thrive in dry, arid regions.
- **Foraging**: Neem trees are common across sub-Saharan Africa, and their leaves, bark, and seeds are commonly foraged for medicinal use. Neem leaves can be boiled to make an antibacterial and antifungal wash, while seeds are used to make oil.

Practical Tips for Foraging African Herbs

Foraging for herbs in the wild can be an enriching and sustainable practice, but it is important to do so responsibly to protect both the plants and the environment. Here are some key considerations for foraging African herbs:

1. **Respect Local Ecosystems**: Always forage sustainably, ensuring that plant populations are not endangered or over-harvested. Only harvest what you need and avoid disturbing the natural habitat of the plants.
2. **Know Your Plants**: It's crucial to properly identify any plant before harvesting. Some plants can be toxic or have similar-looking counterparts that are dangerous. Always consult an expert or reference guides before foraging.
3. **Seasonal Harvesting**: Some plants are best harvested at specific times of the year. For example, certain herbs may be most potent when they are in full bloom or during a particular phase of their growth cycle.
4. **Preserve and Store**: Once harvested, most herbs need to be dried or processed before they can be used. Proper drying techniques will ensure that the medicinal properties of the herbs are preserved. Store dried herbs in cool, dry, airtight containers to prevent degradation.

Cultural Connection

The practice of foraging and growing African herbs is deeply tied to the continent's cultural and spiritual traditions. These herbs, rich in medicinal value, serve not only as remedies for physical ailments but also as tools for maintaining a connection with the natural world. By growing and foraging African herbs, individuals can foster a deeper understanding of the land, promote sustainability, and continue the ancient practice of herbal healing.

Whether you are a novice or experienced herbalist, cultivating and foraging African herbs is an enriching journey that offers both health benefits and cultural insight. As you explore the incredible diversity of African herbal medicine, you will discover a wealth of knowledge and wisdom that spans generations, helping you achieve holistic health and well-being.

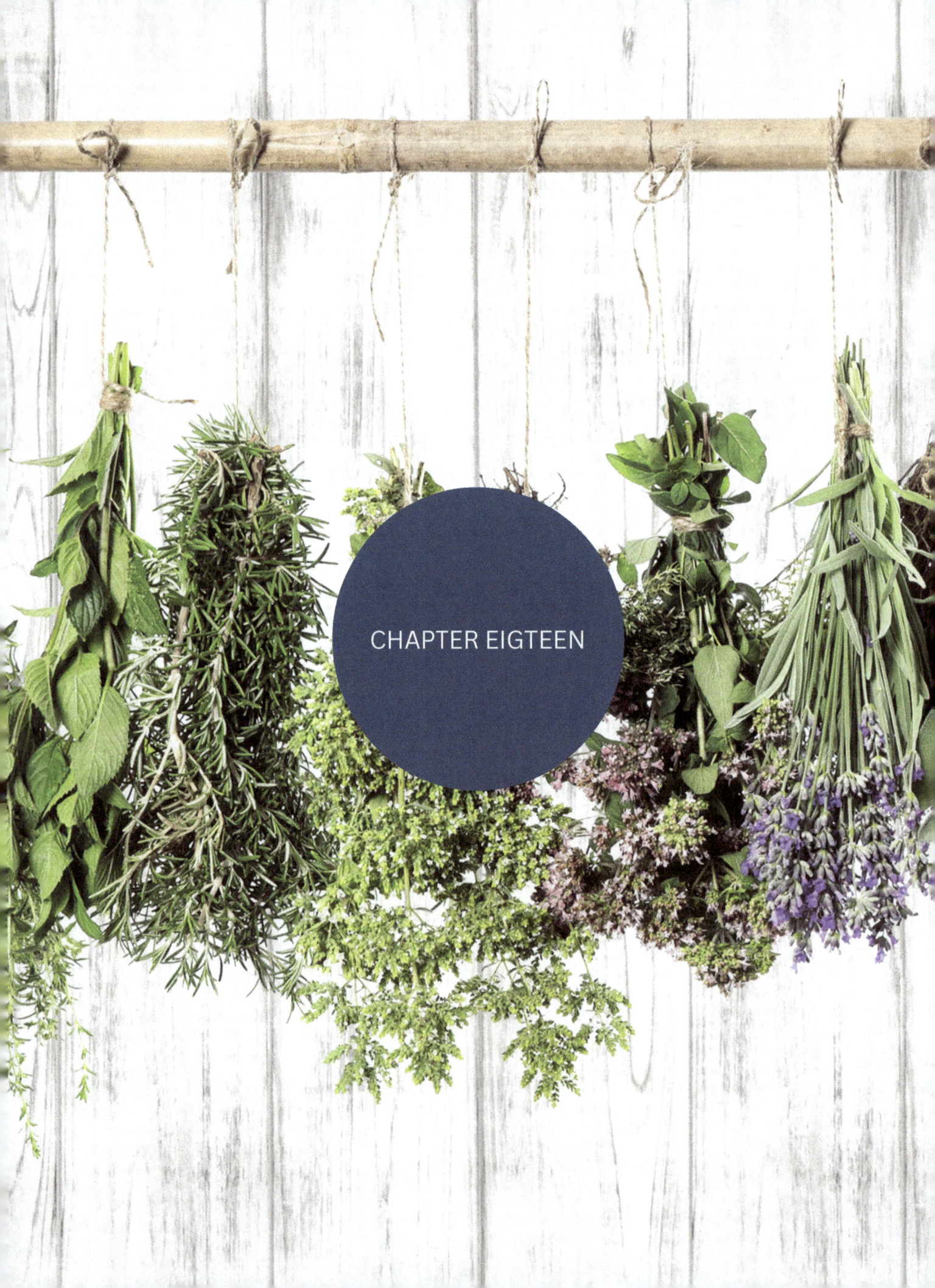

CHAPTER EIGTEEN

The Asian Apothecary

Principles of Traditional Chinese Medicine and Ayurveda

Asia is home to some of the world's oldest and most influential systems of herbal medicine. Among these, Traditional Chinese Medicine (TCM) and Ayurveda stand as two of the most significant, having shaped health practices for thousands of years. Both systems embrace a holistic approach to healing, emphasizing balance, energy flow, and the interconnectedness of the body, mind, and spirit. The principles of these ancient traditions continue to influence modern medicine and herbal practices worldwide.

This chapter explores the core principles of Traditional Chinese Medicine and Ayurveda, focusing on their approach to herbal medicine and the ways in which their practices have been integrated into modern apothecaries.

Traditional Chinese Medicine (TCM)

Traditional Chinese Medicine (TCM) is a medical system that has evolved over more than 2,000 years. It combines herbal medicine, acupuncture, cupping therapy, and other modalities to treat the body, mind, and spirit. TCM is based on the concept of Qi (vital energy) and the balance between the Yin and Yang (the complementary forces of the universe).

Key Concepts in TCM Herbal Medicine:

1. Qi (Vital Energy): Qi is the life force that flows through the body along pathways called meridians. Illness occurs when the flow of Qi is disrupted, either through an excess or deficiency of energy. Herbs in TCM are used to regulate the flow of Qi, restore balance, and improve vitality.
2. Yin and Yang: The concept of Yin and Yang represents the balance of opposites in nature and the body. Yin is associated with coolness, rest, and substance, while Yang represents warmth, activity, and function. Herbs are classified as either Yin or Yang, and the goal of TCM is to maintain or restore harmony between these forces in the body.

1. **Five Elements Theory**: TCM also uses the Five Elements—Wood, Fire, Earth, Metal, and Water—to describe the natural cycles and patterns of the body's systems. Each element corresponds to specific organs, emotions, and seasons, and herbs are selected to nourish and balance these elements.
2. **The Role of the Organs**: In TCM, the organs are not only responsible for physiological functions but also have emotional and spiritual significance. The **Liver**, **Heart**, **Spleen**, **Lungs**, and **Kidneys** are considered the core organs, and each has its associated herbal remedies to support their functioning.

Common Herbs in TCM:
1. **Ginseng (Panax ginseng)**: Known for boosting energy, strengthening immunity, and enhancing mental clarity, ginseng is considered a powerful Yang tonic.
2. **Astragalus (Astragalus membranaceus)**: This herb is used to strengthen the immune system, combat fatigue, and treat respiratory illnesses.
3. **Reishi Mushroom (Ganoderma lucidum)**: Reishi is regarded as a herb of immortality, used for its calming effects, to boost the immune system, and support longevity.
4. **Gingko Biloba (Ginkgo biloba)**: A well-known herb for enhancing cognitive function, particularly memory and focus.
5. **Schisandra (Schisandra chinensis)**: Used to balance Qi, improve energy, and enhance endurance.

Ayurveda

Ayurveda, the traditional medicine system of India, is one of the oldest and most comprehensive systems of herbal healing. It translates to the "science of life" (Ayur = life, Veda = science) and focuses on maintaining balance in the body's three Doshas—Vata, Pitta, and Kapha. These Doshas are believed to govern the physical, mental, and emotional processes of an individual.

Key Concepts in Ayurveda Herbal Medicine:

1. The Three Doshas: The Doshas are unique combinations of the five elements (earth, water, fire, air, and ether) and represent different aspects of human physiology and personality. The Doshas govern various bodily functions, and maintaining their balance is central to good health.
   - Vata: Comprised of Air and Ether, Vata governs movement, circulation, and the nervous system. Imbalances often manifest as dryness, anxiety, and irregular digestion.
   - Pitta: Comprised of Fire and Water, Pitta governs metabolism, digestion, and transformation. Imbalances can lead to inflammation, anger, and digestive issues.
   - Kapha: Comprised of Earth and Water, Kapha governs structure, stability, and lubrication in the body. Imbalances result in lethargy, weight gain, and congestion.
2. Prakriti (Constitution): Each person has a unique combination of the three Doshas, which is referred to as their Prakriti. Understanding your Prakriti helps to tailor treatments, including herbal remedies, for optimal health.

The Five Elements: Just as in TCM, Ayurveda views the body as being influenced by the five elements. Herbs are classified according to the elements they represent and are used to balance the elements within the body.

1. **Agni (Digestive Fire)**: In Ayurveda, **Agni** refers to the digestive fire that governs digestion and metabolism. A strong Agni is essential for health, and many Ayurvedic herbs are used to improve digestive function and restore balance to the body's metabolism.
2. **Ojas (Vital Essence)**: Ojas represents the body's energy reserves and vitality. It is considered essential for immunity, strength, and mental clarity. Herbs are used in Ayurveda to enhance Ojas and promote overall well-being.

Common Herbs in Ayurveda:
1. **Ashwagandha (Withania somnifera)**: Known as a powerful adaptogen, Ashwagandha is used to reduce stress, improve energy, and enhance overall vitality.
2. **Turmeric (Curcuma longa)**: Widely known for its anti-inflammatory and antioxidant properties, turmeric supports digestion, joint health, and skin vitality.
3. **Tulsi (Ocimum sanctum)**: Also called Holy Basil, Tulsi is revered for its immune-boosting, stress-relieving, and anti-inflammatory effects.
4. **Triphala**: A combination of three fruits—Amalaki (Indian gooseberry), Bibhitaki, and Haritaki—Triphala is used as a digestive tonic, cleansing the body and rejuvenating the digestive system.

Neem (Azadirachta indica): In Ayurveda, neem is valued for its detoxifying and antibacterial properties. It is used to purify the blood, treat skin conditions, and strengthen the immune system

Integration of TCM and Ayurveda in Modern Herbal Medicine

Both Traditional Chinese Medicine and Ayurveda have experienced significant globalization in recent years, influencing modern herbal practices worldwide. Their principles emphasize personalized care, a holistic view of the body, and an understanding of the body's natural rhythm and balance.

1. Holistic Health: Both systems treat the root cause of ailments, rather than just addressing symptoms. For example, in TCM, imbalances in Qi or Yin-Yang can lead to illness, while in Ayurveda, an imbalance in the Doshas causes disease. Modern herbal medicine can integrate these insights, offering a comprehensive approach to healing.
2. Herbal Synergy: Many modern herbalists use a combination of herbs from both TCM and Ayurveda to enhance the healing process. For instance, combining Ginseng (from TCM) with Ashwagandha (from Ayurveda) may help to balance energy levels while supporting stress management and overall vitality.
3. Preventive Medicine: Both traditions emphasize prevention and self-care. Herbs are used not only for treating illness but also for maintaining health and preventing future diseases. Modern herbalists often use these principles to create wellness protocols that incorporate herbs for both healing and long-term health maintenance.

Combining Ancient and Modern Herbal Wisdom

Europe's rich and diverse history of herbalism spans thousands of years, shaped by ancient civilizations, monastic traditions, and modern scientific discoveries. From the classical herbal remedies of the ancient Greeks and Romans to the sophisticated botanical studies of the Renaissance, Europe has long been a center of herbal knowledge and healing. Today, the European apothecary combines these ancient practices with cutting-edge research, creating a unique fusion of old and new wisdom.

This chapter explores the foundations of European herbalism, from its ancient origins to its contemporary practices. It examines how ancient knowledge has been preserved, refined, and integrated into modern apothecaries, and how this blend continues to inspire modern herbal medicine.

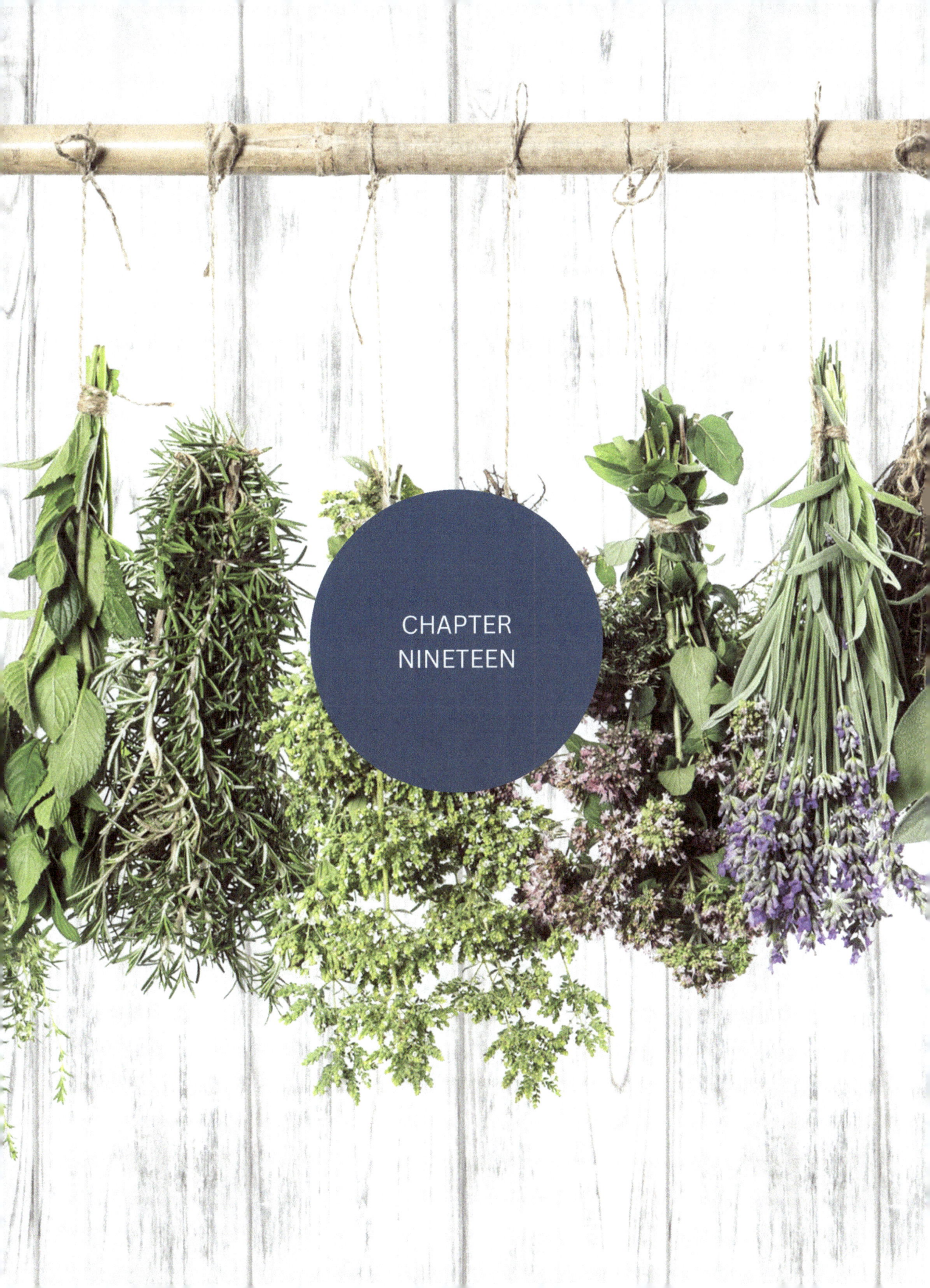

CHAPTER NINETEEN

The Foundations of European Herbal Medicine

European herbal traditions are deeply rooted in the civilizations of ancient Greece and Rome. Early herbalism in Europe was a blend of local traditions, including the use of indigenous plants for healing, and influences from the far reaches of the ancient world, such as Egypt and Mesopotamia. These civilizations laid the foundation for what would later become Western herbalism.

Ancient Greece and Rome

Hippocrates, often referred to as the "Father of Medicine," advocated for the use of natural remedies, including herbs, to maintain health and treat disease. His teachings on the balance of the four humors (blood, phlegm, yellow bile, and black bile) shaped early European medical thought.

Dioscorides, a Greek physician, is renowned for his work De Materia Medica, a comprehensive herbal text that cataloged over 600 plants and their medicinal properties. This text became the cornerstone of European herbal medicine for centuries.

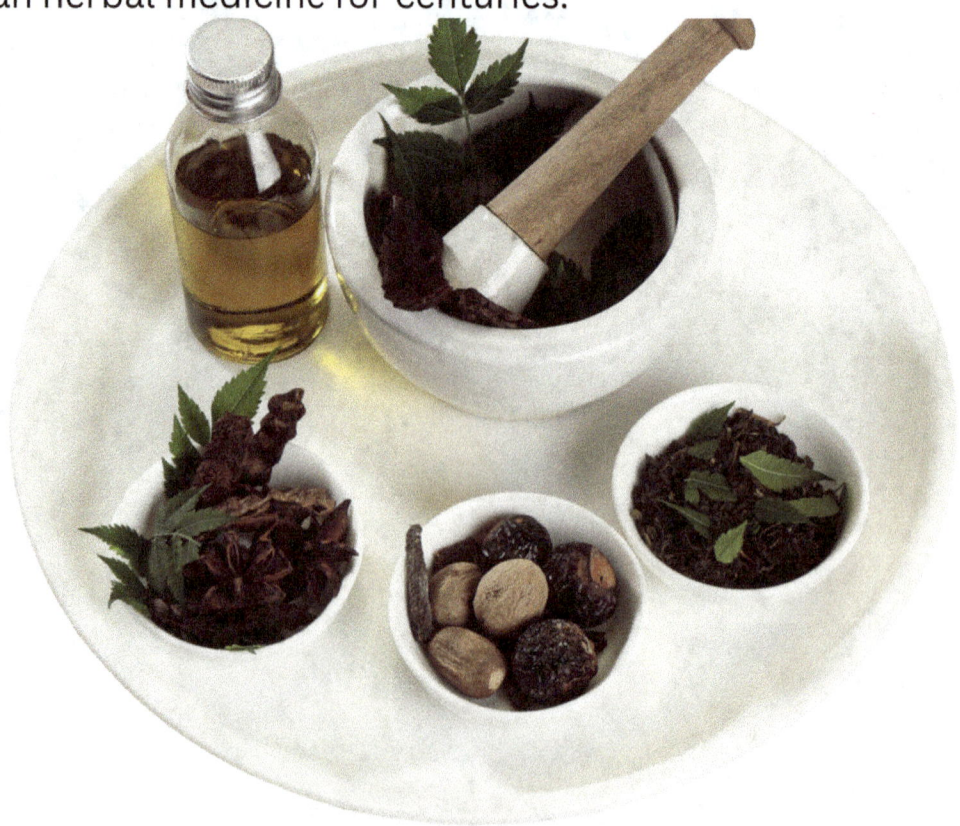

- **Pliny the Elder**, a Roman author and naturalist, wrote *Natural History*, which included detailed descriptions of medicinal plants used by the Romans and others, influencing later herbal texts.

Medieval and Renaissance Europe

- During the Middle Ages, the church played a key role in preserving and transmitting herbal knowledge. **Monasteries** became centers of learning where monks carefully cultivated medicinal plants in their gardens and produced herbal remedies for the sick. Many of these traditions are still practiced today in modern European apothecaries.
- The **Renaissance** saw a revival of interest in classical texts and the study of plants. Botanists like **Paracelsus** and **Nicholas Culpeper** advanced herbal knowledge, combining traditional remedies with new insights into the chemical properties of plants. Culpeper's *Complete Herbal* remains one of the most widely used herbals in the Western tradition.

The Modern European Apothecary

In modern times, European herbal medicine has evolved into a sophisticated system of practice that combines ancient knowledge with modern scientific understanding. The rise of **phytotherapy**, or the use of plant-based medicines, has been a key development in the 19th and 20th centuries, as new methods of extracting and isolating plant compounds led to a more precise understanding of their therapeutic effects.

Phytotherapy and the Scientific Approach

- Phytotherapy is the study and use of plant-derived medications to treat illness. In Europe, phytotherapy is a well-established branch of medicine and is often used in conjunction with conventional treatments. The effectiveness of many herbal remedies is now backed by scientific research, which has identified active compounds in plants that are responsible for their healing properties.
- Herbs such as St. John's Wort, Elderberry, Chamomile, and Lavender are now widely recognized for their medicinal value, with studies confirming their efficacy in treating conditions like depression, respiratory infections, and digestive issues.

Herbal Medicine in European Pharmacies

In Europe, particularly in countries like Germany, France, and Switzerland, herbal remedies are integrated into mainstream healthcare. Germany, for instance, has a long tradition of using herbal monographs—official documents that list the therapeutic uses, safety information, and dosage of medicinal plants.

- Germany has a robust system of regulation for herbal products, with agencies like the Commission E providing guidance on the safety and efficacy of plant-based medicines.
- France has its own tradition of herbal medicine, with many herbs used to support daily wellness, such as Tisanes (herbal teas) and Fleurs de Bach remedies (flower essences).

Key Herbs in the European Apothecary

European herbalism emphasizes the importance of using herbs for both prevention and treatment of illnesses. These herbs are typically used in teas, tinctures, oils, and ointments. Some of the most commonly used herbs in the European apothecary include:

1. Lavender (Lavandula angustifolia):
   - Uses: Lavender is widely known for its calming and relaxing effects. It is commonly used to treat anxiety, insomnia, headaches, and skin irritations.
   - Modern Applications: In aromatherapy, lavender essential oil is used to reduce stress and improve sleep quality. It is also used in topical applications for minor burns, insect bites, and skin rashes.
2. Chamomile (Matricaria chamomilla):
   - Uses: Chamomile has been used for centuries for its soothing properties, especially for digestive issues like indigestion, bloating, and colic.
   - Modern Applications: Chamomile tea remains a popular remedy for insomnia and anxiety. It is also used topically in ointments to soothe skin conditions such as eczema or minor cuts.
3. St. John's Wort (Hypericum perforatum):
   - Uses: Traditionally used for its mood-enhancing properties, St. John's Wort is well-known for its ability to alleviate mild to moderate depression.
   - Modern Applications: Clinical research has validated its effectiveness for treating depression, and it is now a popular supplement in many countries.
4. Elderberry (Sambucus nigra):
   - Uses: Elderberry has a long history of use in Europe, particularly for boosting the immune system and treating colds and flu.
   - Modern Applications: Elderberry syrups and lozenges are widely used to shorten the duration and severity of cold and flu symptoms. It is rich in antioxidants and vitamins that support immune function.

1. **Thyme (Thymus vulgaris)**:
   - **Uses**: Thyme is a powerful herb used to treat respiratory issues like coughs, bronchitis, and asthma. It is also a natural antiseptic.
   - **Modern Applications**: Thyme essential oil is used in steam inhalations to clear respiratory passages and as an ingredient in chest rubs for colds.
2. **Nettle (Urtica dioica)**:
   - **Uses**: Nettle has been used for centuries to treat joint pain, allergies, and urinary tract problems. It is considered a strong tonic for the kidneys and urinary system.
   - **Modern Applications**: Nettle is used in herbal teas, capsules, and tinctures to support detoxification, reduce inflammation, and promote overall vitality.

Integrating Ancient and Modern Approaches

The European apothecary is unique in its ability to combine traditional knowledge with scientific validation. Modern herbalists in Europe often blend ancient practices with the latest findings from botanical research to create effective remedies that are both time-tested and scientifically proven.

Synergy Between Traditional and Modern Wisdom

- Ancient herbal texts, such as those written by Dioscorides and Culpeper, provide valuable insights into the healing properties of plants that modern science is now able to investigate further. This synergy between ancient knowledge and modern research allows herbal medicine to thrive in a contemporary context.
- Modern herbalists continue to use the same techniques for making herbal preparations (teas, tinctures, infusions), while incorporating advanced methods of extraction and formulation that enhance the potency and bioavailability of plant compounds.

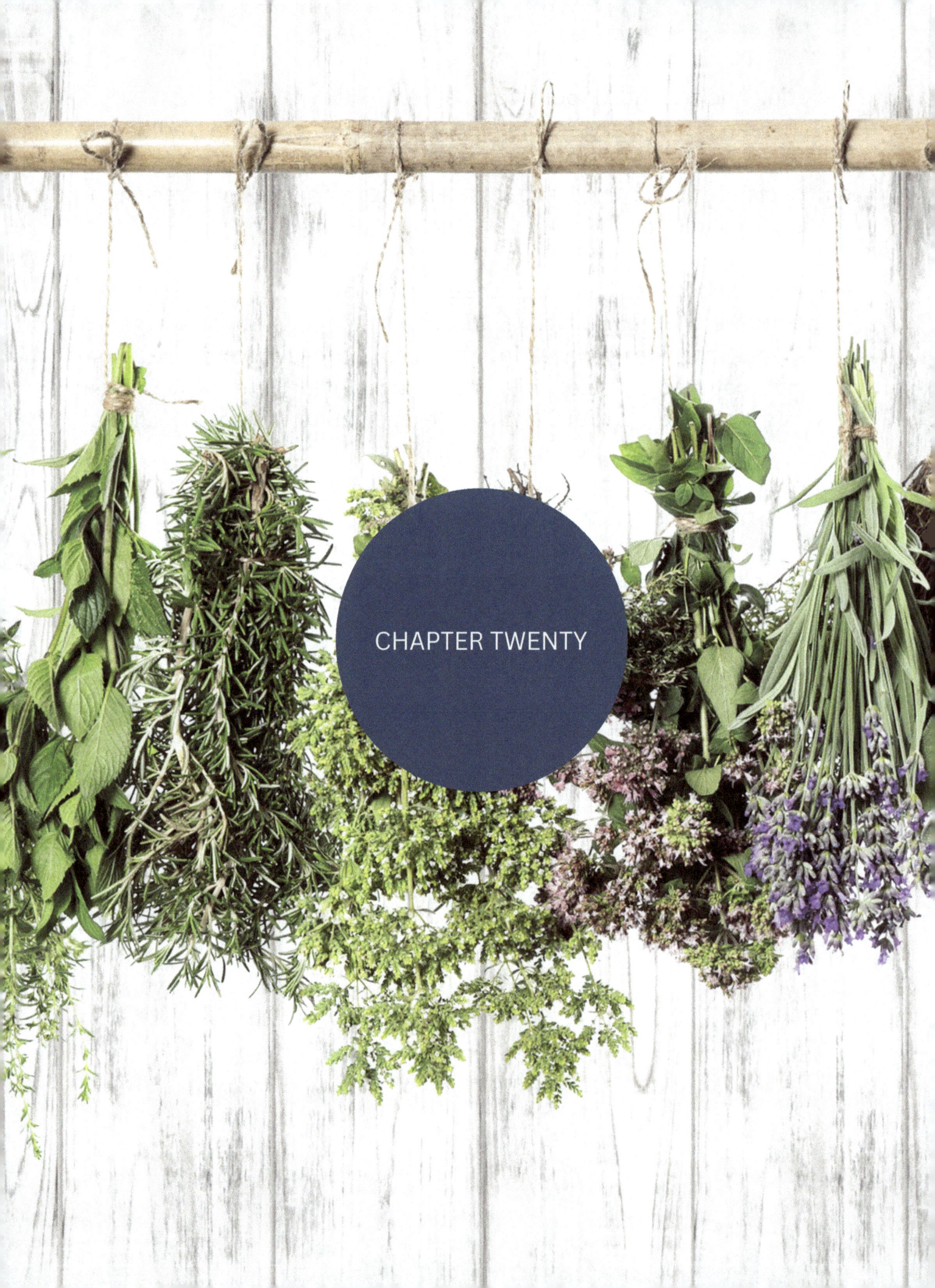

CHAPTER TWENTY

The Americas' Apothecary: Sacred Healing Practices from Indigenous Communities

The Americas, a vast continent with rich cultural diversity, is home to a wide array of indigenous healing traditions. From the temperate forests of North America to the jungles of the Amazon in South America, indigenous communities have long relied on the natural world for medicinal practices. For thousands of years, these traditions have been based on a deep, spiritual connection to the earth, respecting the plants, animals, and elements that sustain life. This chapter explores the sacred healing practices of indigenous communities in the Americas, focusing on their use of native plants, spiritual guidance, and holistic approaches to wellness.

Sacred Connection to the Land

For indigenous peoples of the Americas, the relationship with nature is not just practical but spiritual. Plants, animals, and natural resources are considered sacred and are regarded as living beings with their own spirits. The healing practices passed down through generations are rooted in a profound respect for the environment and the belief that everything in nature is interconnected.

This spiritual connection forms the foundation of traditional indigenous healing systems, where herbal medicine, rituals, ceremonies, and prayers are all intertwined. Healers, known by various names such as shamans, medicine men and women, and herbalists, are often considered intermediaries between the physical and spiritual worlds. Their knowledge of plant medicine and healing rituals is passed down through oral traditions and often carries deep symbolic and cultural significance.

Key Herbs of the Americas' Apothecary

Indigenous healing practices across the Americas use a variety of herbs that are native to the regions, each with its own unique healing properties. These plants are utilized not only for their medicinal properties but also in ceremonies and rituals that are integral to the culture of indigenous peoples.

North America: Sacred Plants of Native Tribes

1. Echinacea (Echinacea purpurea)
   - Uses: Echinacea is one of the most well-known herbs in North America, particularly in the United States, where it has been used by many Native American tribes, such as the Lakota, for immune support and to treat infections. It is considered a powerful immune stimulant.
   - Traditional Uses: Native American healers would use Echinacea as a tonic for general health, treating colds, wounds, and sore throats.
   - Modern Applications: Echinacea is commonly used today as a natural remedy for colds, flu, and other respiratory infections, and is available in tinctures, teas, and capsules.
2. Sage (Salvia spp.)
   - Uses: Sage holds immense spiritual and medicinal significance in many Native American cultures. White sage, in particular, is used in purification ceremonies (smudging), where its smoke is believed to cleanse the body, mind, and spirit.
   - Traditional Uses: Native American tribes like the Navajo, Hopi, and Lakota use sage to cleanse spaces of negative energy and as a healing herb for colds, coughs, and digestive issues.
   - Modern Applications: In addition to its use in smudging rituals, sage is commonly consumed in teas and tinctures for its antibacterial properties and its role in digestive health.

3. **Willow Bark (Salix spp.)**
    - **Uses**: Willow bark has long been used by Native American tribes as a remedy for pain, particularly for headaches, back pain, and menstrual cramps. It contains **salicin**, a compound chemically similar to aspirin.
    - **Traditional Uses**: Native Americans would brew willow bark tea to reduce pain and inflammation and used it as a treatment for fevers.
    - **Modern Applications**: Willow bark is still used today in herbal medicine for its natural analgesic and anti-inflammatory effects.
4. **Yarrow (Achillea millefolium)**
    - **Uses**: Yarrow is revered by many North American tribes for its ability to heal wounds and reduce bleeding. It has been traditionally used as a poultice for cuts and injuries.
    - **Traditional Uses**: Native Americans used yarrow for wound healing, to stop bleeding, and as a remedy for colds, fevers, and digestive issues.
    - **Modern Applications**: Yarrow is still utilized in modern herbalism for its antibacterial, anti-inflammatory, and astringent properties.
5, **Sweetgrass (Hierochloe odorata)**
    - **Uses**: Sweetgrass is considered sacred in many Native American cultures, often used in ceremonial rituals and for spiritual purification. It is believed to have protective qualities.
    - **Traditional Uses**: Native American tribes like the Cree and the Ojibwe use sweetgrass to make braided offerings for sacred spaces, as well as to promote healing, peace, and positive energy.
    - **Modern Applications**: Sweetgrass is used in herbal preparations for calming and soothing, and its smoke is still commonly used in smudging ceremonies.

South America: Sacred Herbs from the Amazon and Beyond

1. Chanca Piedra (Phyllanthus niruri)
   - Uses: Known as the "stone breaker," Chanca Piedra is highly valued in indigenous Amazonian medicine for its ability to treat kidney stones, gallstones, and urinary tract infections.
   - Traditional Uses: Indigenous tribes in the Amazon have used Chanca Piedra for centuries to treat kidney issues and cleanse the urinary tract.
   - Modern Applications: Chanca Piedra is now studied for its anti-lithiasis properties, with growing interest in its use for kidney stone prevention and treatment.
2. Guarana (Paullinia cupana)
   - Uses: Guarana is a potent stimulant that is used to improve energy, mental focus, and physical stamina. It is traditionally used by tribes in the Amazon as an energizing herb.
   - Traditional Uses: Indigenous groups like the Satere-Mawe use guarana seeds to create a drink that provides increased energy and stamina, especially for physical labor.
   - Modern Applications: Guarana is widely used in energy drinks, supplements, and weight loss products for its stimulating effects.
3. Yerba Mate (Ilex paraguariensis)
   - Uses: Yerba Mate is a traditional herbal tea widely consumed in South American countries like Argentina, Paraguay, and Brazil. It is known for its stimulating effects, thanks to its caffeine content.
   - Traditional Uses: Indigenous peoples of the Guarani tribe in Paraguay and Argentina have been drinking yerba mate for centuries, using it for its energizing properties, as well as for digestive and immune support.
   - Modern Applications: Yerba mate is popular worldwide as an alternative to coffee and is available in various forms, including teas, powders, and capsules.

4., **Achiote (Bixa orellana)**
    - **Uses**: Known for its vibrant red seeds, achiote is a traditional herb used by Amazonian tribes for its anti-inflammatory and antioxidant properties.
    - **Traditional Uses**: The seeds of achiote are used in traditional herbal remedies to treat inflammation, improve skin health, and boost immunity.
    - **Modern Applications**: Achiote is used in modern herbalism to support skin health and provide antioxidants that promote overall wellness.
5. **Quinine (Cinchona officinalis)**
    - **Uses**: Quinine, derived from the bark of the cinchona tree, has been used for centuries by indigenous communities in South America to treat malaria and fevers.
    - **Traditional Uses**: Indigenous tribes in the Andes used quinine to treat fevers and malaria, as well as to alleviate pain and digestive issues.
    - **Modern Applications**: Quinine remains a crucial ingredient in the treatment of malaria and is still used in modern medicine for its antimalarial properties.

Spiritual and Ritual Healing

Indigenous apothecaries are not limited to the use of physical herbs; spiritual and ceremonial practices are essential components of healing. For many tribes, healing is a holistic experience that integrates mind, body, and spirit. In these cultures, plants are often used in conjunction with rituals, prayers, and ceremonies to invoke spiritual protection, purification, and healing.

- Sacred Ceremonies: In many indigenous cultures, sacred herbs are used in rituals designed to call upon ancestral spirits, the forces of nature, and divine energies. These ceremonies are thought to facilitate the healing process by restoring balance to the body, mind, and spirit.
- Shamanic Practices: Shamans or spiritual healers use sacred plants in rituals to communicate with spirits, diagnose illness, and restore health. This often involves the use of ayahuasca, a powerful plant-based brew used by Amazonian tribes, which is considered a spiritual medicine that can provide visions and insight into a person's condition.

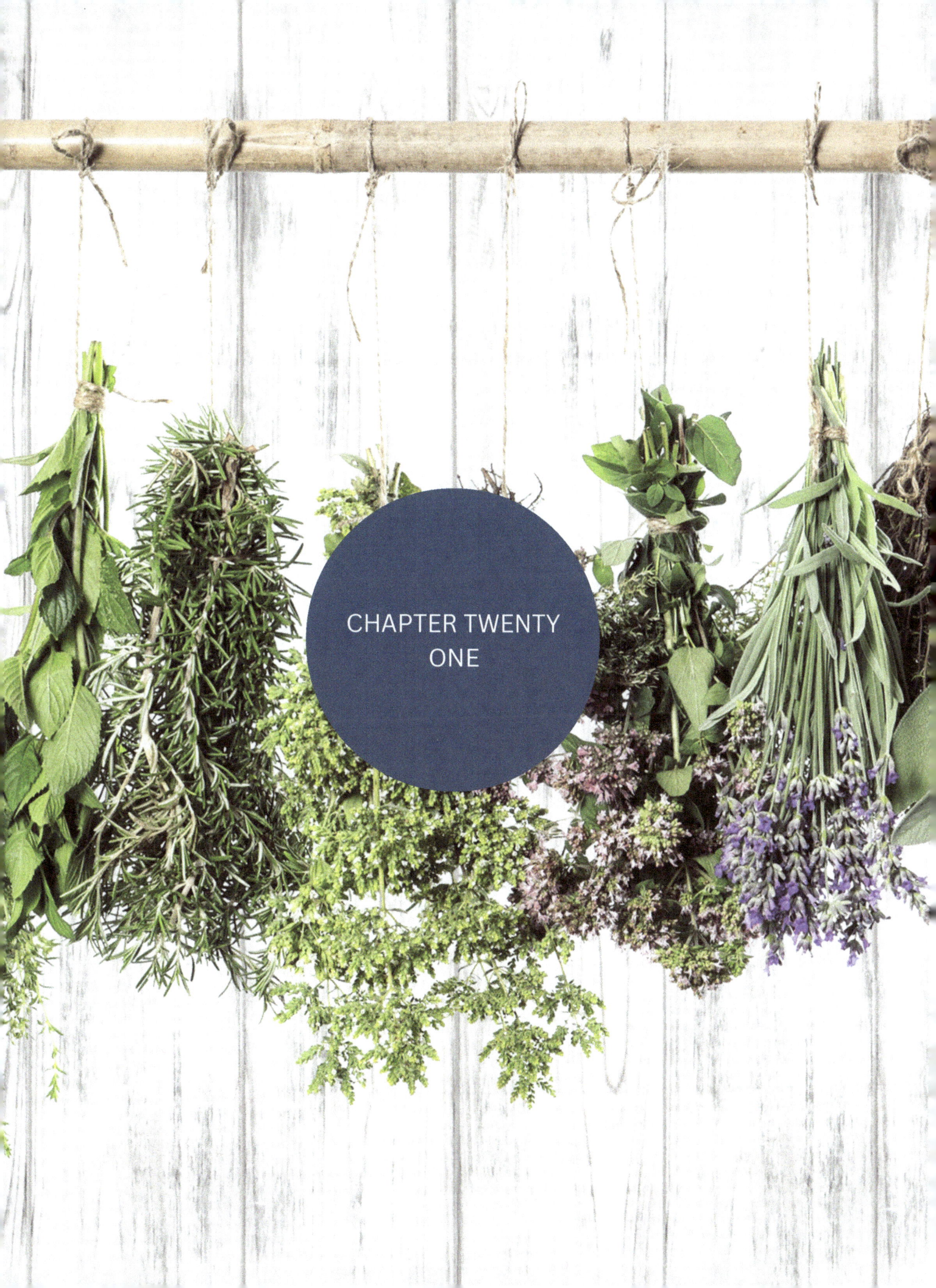

CHAPTER TWENTY ONE

The Island Apothecary: Polynesian and Oceanic Healing Secrets

Polynesia and Oceania, with their stunning landscapes of tropical islands and expansive seas, are home to vibrant traditions of natural medicine. Rooted in a deep connection to nature and the cycles of life, Polynesian and Oceanic healing secrets have been preserved through oral traditions, storytelling, and rituals passed down over generations. The island apothecaries of these regions harness the power of native plants, marine resources, and holistic practices to address physical, mental, and spiritual well-being.

Foundations of Polynesian and Oceanic Healing

Island cultures view health and healing as a harmonious balance between the individual, community, and environment. This belief system underpins the holistic approaches employed in traditional Polynesian and Oceanic medicine. Some core principles include:

1. Mana (Life Energy): Mana is a spiritual force believed to exist in all living things. In Polynesian healing traditions, maintaining or restoring mana is essential for health and vitality. Rituals and remedies often aim to restore balance to an individual's mana.
2. Holistic Wellness: Health is seen as a state of balance encompassing the body, mind, and spirit. Healers focus on addressing the root cause of ailments rather than just symptoms, incorporating physical remedies, spiritual rituals, and communal support.
3. Connection to Nature: The abundance of natural resources on the islands—plants, trees, fruits, and even marine life—forms the basis of traditional apothecaries. Islanders have developed an intimate understanding of their environment, using local resources for both food and medicine.

Key Healing Plants of the Polynesian and Oceanic Traditions

Island apothecaries are rich with a variety of plants renowned for their medicinal and therapeutic properties. These herbs and remedies are used to treat common ailments, strengthen the body, and promote longevity.

1. Kava (Piper methysticum)
- Uses: Revered across the Pacific Islands, kava is used for its calming effects. It is known for relieving stress, anxiety, and insomnia, and for promoting relaxation and social bonding.
- Traditional Applications: Kava root is prepared as a ceremonial drink, often consumed during rituals to foster peace and connection. It is also used as a mild sedative and muscle relaxant.
- Modern Applications: Kava is now recognized globally as a natural remedy for anxiety and is available in capsules, teas, and extracts.

2. Noni (Morinda citrifolia)
- Uses: Known as the "Queen of Polynesian Medicine," noni is prized for its immune-boosting and anti-inflammatory properties. It is used to treat skin conditions, infections, and digestive issues.
- Traditional Applications: The fruit, leaves, and roots of the noni plant are used in poultices, teas, and topical preparations. Islanders often drink fermented noni juice for its detoxifying and healing benefits.
- Modern Applications: Noni is marketed as a superfood, with juices and supplements widely available for supporting immune health and overall wellness.

3. Breadfruit Leaves (Artocarpus altilis)
- **Uses**: While breadfruit is a staple food in Polynesia, its leaves have medicinal properties, particularly for managing blood sugar levels and supporting cardiovascular health.
- **Traditional Applications**: Breadfruit leaves are brewed into teas to help with diabetes, high blood pressure, and skin conditions.
- **Modern Applications**: Breadfruit leaf tea is gaining recognition as a natural remedy for metabolic and cardiovascular disorders.

4. Ti Leaf (Cordyline fruticosa)
- **Uses**: Ti leaves are versatile in their applications, often used for protection, purification, and wound healing.
- **Traditional Applications**: In Polynesian culture, ti leaves are woven into leis, wrapped around injuries, or used in steam baths for their cleansing properties.
- **Modern Applications**: Ti leaf extracts are included in wellness products for their soothing and anti-inflammatory effects.

5. Kukui Nut (Aleurites moluccanus)
- **Uses**: The kukui nut tree, also known as the candlenut tree, is revered for its skin-nourishing properties. It is used to treat dry skin, sunburns, and wounds.
- **Traditional Applications**: Kukui nut oil is extracted and applied topically to hydrate and heal the skin. It is also used in massage therapies for its soothing effects.
- **Modern Applications**: Kukui nut oil is a popular ingredient in skincare products, especially for moisturizing and repairing damaged skin.

Rituals and Spiritual Healing

In Polynesian and Oceanic cultures, healing is deeply intertwined with spirituality. Rituals and ceremonies are vital to restoring harmony and balance, both within the individual and in their relationship with the community and nature.

1. Lomilomi Massage:
   - A traditional Hawaiian healing practice, lomilomi incorporates rhythmic massage, prayer (pule), and meditation to release tension, improve circulation, and balance the body's energy.
2. Rongoā Māori:
   - In Māori culture of New Zealand, rongoā is a traditional healing system involving herbal remedies, spiritual guidance, and massage therapies. Practitioners, known as tohunga, work to heal both physical and spiritual ailments.
3. Firewalking and Ceremonial Dances:
   - Some island communities perform firewalking rituals or ceremonial dances to invoke blessings, promote healing, and cleanse negative energy.
4. Seawater Therapy:
   - The ocean itself is considered a source of healing. Bathing in seawater or using seawater in treatments is believed to cleanse the body, improve circulation, and promote relaxation.

Herbal Preparations and Uses

Traditional Polynesian and Oceanic apothecaries often use simple yet effective preparation methods to harness the power of their native plants.

- Teas and Decoctions: Herbal teas are commonly prepared from leaves, roots, and bark. For example, kava tea is consumed for relaxation, while breadfruit leaf tea supports metabolic health.
- Poultices and Salves: Crushed herbs like noni leaves or kukui nuts are applied directly to wounds or skin conditions to promote healing.
- Oils and Infusions: Kukui nut oil and coconut oil are infused with other healing herbs for use in massages and topical treatments.

Modern Applications and Global Recognition

The healing traditions of Polynesia and Oceania have gained international attention for their natural remedies and holistic approaches. Many island herbs, such as kava and noni, are now staples in the global wellness market. Modern science continues to study these traditional remedies, validating their efficacy and expanding their reach.

Preserving Island Wisdom

As interest in traditional Polynesian and Oceanic medicine grows, it is crucial to respect and preserve the cultural and spiritual heritage of these healing practices. Collaborations between indigenous healers and modern researchers can ensure the continuation of these traditions while safeguarding their integrity.

By embracing the wisdom of the Island Apothecary, we can learn to integrate the harmony of nature into our own lives, fostering wellness that goes beyond the physical and touches the spirit.

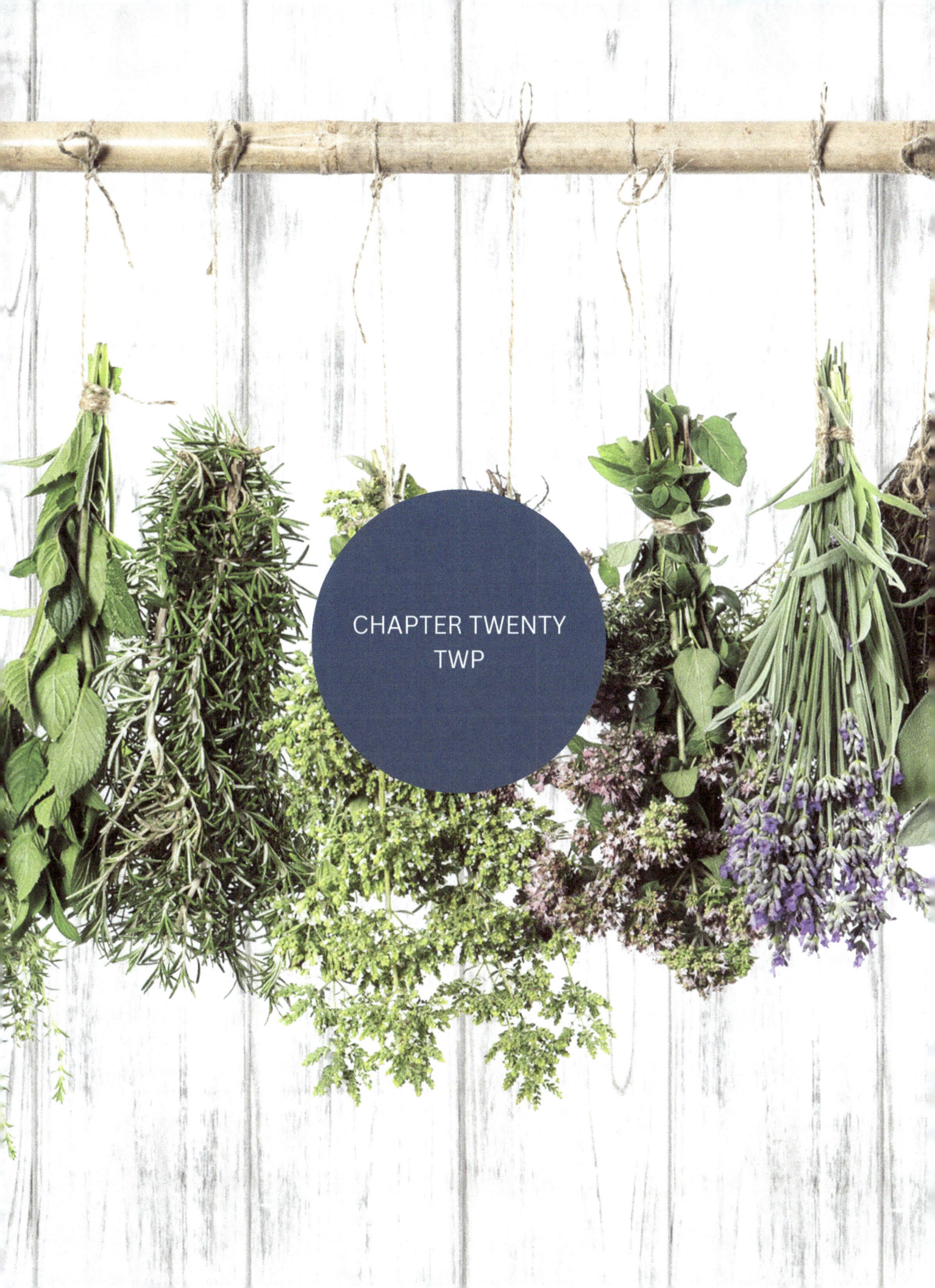

CHAPTER TWENTY TWP

Herbal Beauty and Self-Care: Skin and Hair Care Recipes

Herbs have been celebrated for centuries as nature's remedy for glowing skin, healthy hair, and overall well-being. Whether used in ancient rituals or modern self-care routines, herbal ingredients offer gentle yet effective solutions that nourish, protect, and enhance natural beauty. These DIY recipes harness the power of botanicals to create luxurious, chemical-free skincare and haircare treatments you can enjoy at home.

Herbal Skincare Recipes
1. Calming Chamomile and Aloe Vera Face Mask
   - Benefits: Soothes sensitive skin, reduces redness, and hydrates.
   - Ingredients:
     a. 1 tablespoon chamomile tea (brewed and cooled)
     b. 2 tablespoons aloe vera gel
     c. 1 teaspoon honey
   - Instructions:
     d. Mix chamomile tea with aloe vera gel and honey.
     e. Apply evenly to your face and neck.
     f. Leave on for 15–20 minutes, then rinse with lukewarm water.
   - Why it works: Chamomile is anti-inflammatory, aloe vera hydrates and soothes, and honey has antibacterial properties.

2. Lavender and Oatmeal Exfoliating Scrub
- **Benefits**: Gently exfoliates dead skin cells and calms irritated skin.
- **Ingredients**:
    a. 1/2 cup ground oatmeal
    b. 2 tablespoons almond oil
    c. 5 drops lavender essential oil
- **Instructions**:
    d. Combine the ingredients in a bowl until you have a thick paste.
    e. Massage gently onto damp skin in circular motions.
    f. Rinse thoroughly with warm water.
- **Why it works**: Oatmeal soothes and exfoliates, almond oil moisturizes, and lavender essential oil calms the skin.

3. Rosehip and Hibiscus Toner
- **Benefits**: Brightens the skin and minimizes pores.
- **Ingredients**:
    a. 1 cup hibiscus tea (brewed and cooled)
    b. 1 teaspoon rosehip oil
    c. 1 tablespoon witch hazel
- **Instructions**:
    d. Mix all the ingredients in a spray bottle.
    e. Shake well and spritz onto your face after cleansing.
- **Why it works**: Hibiscus is rich in antioxidants, rosehip oil rejuvenates, and witch hazel tones the skin.

4. Neem and Turmeric Spot Treatment

- **Benefits**: Treats acne and prevents future breakouts.
- **Ingredients**:
    a. 1/2 teaspoon neem powder
    b. 1/4 teaspoon turmeric powder
    c. 1 teaspoon water
- **Instructions**:
    d. Mix the powders with water to form a paste.
    e. Apply to blemishes and leave on for 10–15 minutes.
    f. Rinse with warm water.
- **Why it works**: Neem is antibacterial, and turmeric reduces inflammation.

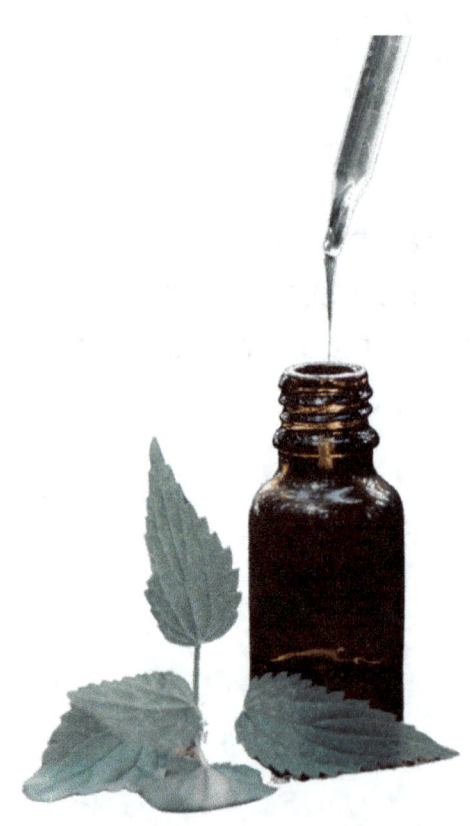

Herbal Hair Care Recipes

1. Rosemary and Peppermint Hair Growth Oil
   - Benefits: Stimulates hair follicles and promotes growth.
   - Ingredients:
     a. 1/4 cup coconut oil
     b. 5 drops rosemary essential oil
     c. 3 drops peppermint essential oil
   - Instructions:
     d. Warm the coconut oil slightly and mix in the essential oils.
     e. Massage into your scalp for 5–10 minutes.
     f. Leave on for at least an hour (or overnight), then shampoo as usual.
   - Why it works: Rosemary improves circulation, and peppermint invigorates the scalp.

2. Hibiscus and Coconut Deep Conditioning Mask
   - Benefits: Restores shine and moisture to dull hair.
   - Ingredients:
     a. 1/2 cup coconut milk
     b. 2 tablespoons hibiscus powder
     c. 1 tablespoon honey
   - Instructions:
     d. Blend all ingredients until smooth.
     e. Apply to damp hair, focusing on the ends.
     f. Cover with a shower cap and leave on for 30 minutes, then rinse thoroughly.
   - Why it works: Hibiscus strengthens hair, coconut milk hydrates, and honey locks in moisture.

3. Nettle and Apple Cider Vinegar Rinse
- **Benefits**: Reduces dandruff and balances scalp pH.
- **Ingredients**:
  a. 2 cups nettle tea (brewed and cooled)
  b. 1/4 cup apple cider vinegar
- **Instructions**:
  c. Combine the tea and vinegar in a jug.
  d. Pour over your scalp and hair after shampooing.
  e. Let it sit for a few minutes, then rinse with cool water.
- **Why it works**: Nettle soothes the scalp, and apple cider vinegar clarifies.

4. Amla and Fenugreek Hair Strengthening Mask
- **Benefits**: Prevents hair breakage and improves elasticity.
- **Ingredients**:
  a. 2 tablespoons amla powder
  b. 1 tablespoon fenugreek powder
  c. 1/2 cup yogurt
- **Instructions**:
  d. Mix the powders with yogurt to form a thick paste.
  e. Apply to your hair and scalp.
  f. Leave on for 30 minutes, then wash out with a mild shampoo.
- **Why it works**: Amla strengthens hair roots, and fenugreek adds protein and shine.

Herbal Self-Care Tips
1. Herbal Baths:
    - Add dried herbs like lavender, chamomile, or rose petals to your bathwater for a relaxing soak. Combine with Epsom salts and essential oils for added benefits.
2. DIY Herbal Steam:
    - Create a facial steam by adding dried herbs like rosemary, mint, or calendula to a bowl of hot water. Drape a towel over your head and let the steam cleanse and refresh your skin.
3. Herbal Pillow Sprays:
    - Blend lavender and chamomile essential oils with distilled water in a spray bottle to create a calming mist for your linens and pillows.
4. Foot Soaks:
    - Soak tired feet in warm water infused with Epsom salts and herbs like peppermint or eucalyptus for relaxation and odor control.

Why Choose Herbal Beauty?
1. Natural and Non-Toxic: Herbal ingredients are free of harmful chemicals, making them safe for most skin and hair types.
2. Eco-Friendly: Using herbs reduces reliance on synthetic products and packaging, promoting sustainable beauty practices.
3. Customizable: You can tailor recipes to your specific needs, preferences, and available ingredients.

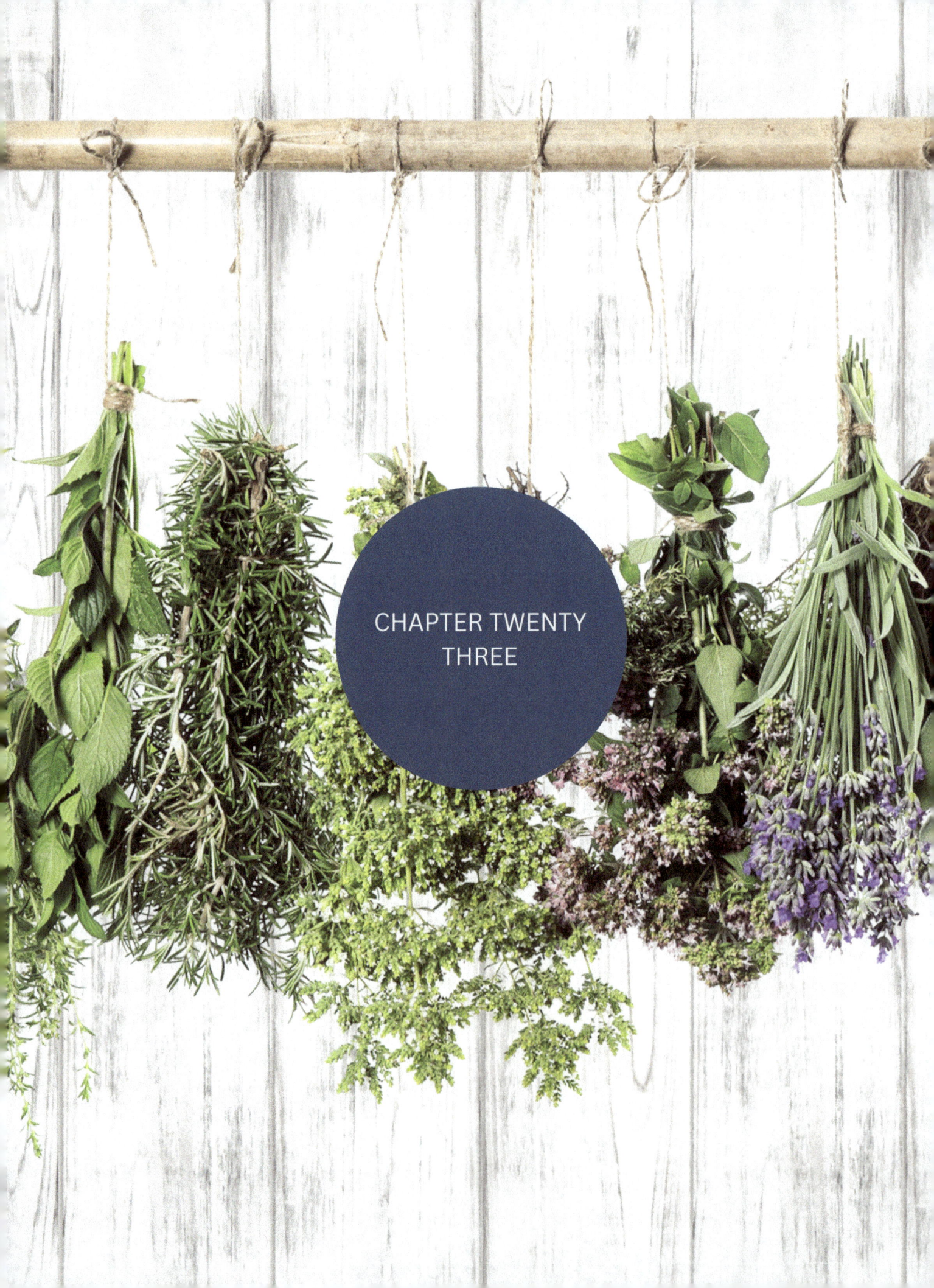

CHAPTER TWENTY THREE

Cooking with Medicinal Herbs

Discover how medicinal herbs can transform everyday meals into nourishing remedies. Across cultures, herbs have been used to enhance flavors while supporting health. This guide explores a variety of global recipes that incorporate healing herbs into delicious and nutritious dishes.

The Role of Medicinal Herbs in Nutrition

Medicinal herbs are packed with bioactive compounds such as antioxidants, vitamins, and minerals that support the body's natural functions. Integrating these herbs into your cooking allows you to enjoy their health benefits in a natural, flavorful way.

Global Recipes with Medicinal Herbs

1. African Moringa Leaf Stew (Nigeria)

- Benefits: Boosts energy, improves digestion, and supports immunity.
- Ingredients:
    a. 2 cups fresh moringa leaves (or 1 cup dried)
    b. 1 cup chopped spinach
    c. 1/2 cup diced tomatoes
    d. 1/4 cup onions, chopped
    e. 1 tablespoon ground crayfish (optional)
    f. 2 tablespoons palm oil
    g. Salt and pepper to taste

- **Instructions**:
    a. Heat palm oil in a pot and sauté onions until translucent.
    b. Add tomatoes and cook until softened.
    c. Stir in moringa leaves, spinach, and ground crayfish.
    d. Simmer for 5–7 minutes, season with salt and pepper, and serve with rice or yams.

2. Asian Turmeric Coconut Rice (India)
- **Benefits**: Reduces inflammation and supports joint health.
- **Ingredients**:
    a. 1 cup basmati rice
    b. 1/2 teaspoon turmeric powder
    c. 1 cup coconut milk
    d. 1 cup water
    e. 1/4 teaspoon black pepper
    f. Salt to taste
- **Instructions**:
    g. Rinse the rice thoroughly and set aside.
    h. In a pot, combine rice, coconut milk, water, turmeric, black pepper, and salt.
    i. Bring to a boil, then reduce heat, cover, and simmer for 15 minutes.
    j. Fluff with a fork and serve with sautéed vegetables or grilled fish.

3. European Lavender-Infused Honey Glaze (France)
- **Benefits**: Promotes relaxation and soothes digestion.
- **Ingredients**:
    a. 1/4 cup honey
    b. 1 teaspoon dried lavender flowers
    c. 1 tablespoon lemon juice
    d. Pinch of salt
- **Instructions**:
    e. Heat honey and lavender in a small saucepan over low heat.
    f. Remove from heat and let steep for 10 minutes.
    g. Strain the lavender, stir in lemon juice and salt, and drizzle over roasted chicken or vegetables.

4. Native American Wild Rice with Sage and Cranberries
- **Benefits**: Supports digestion and provides antioxidants.
- **Ingredients**:
    a. 1 cup wild rice
    b. 2 1/2 cups water or vegetable broth
    c. 1/4 cup dried cranberries
    d. 1 teaspoon dried sage
    e. 1 tablespoon olive oil
    f. Salt and pepper to taste
- **Instructions**:
    g. Rinse wild rice and cook in water or broth according to package instructions.
    h. Toss cooked rice with cranberries, sage, olive oil, and seasoning.
    i. Serve as a side dish with roasted turkey or vegetables.

5. Latin American Cilantro Chimichurri (Argentina)
- **Benefits**: Detoxifies the body and aids digestion.
- **Ingredients**:
    a. 1 cup fresh cilantro leaves
    b. 1/4 cup fresh parsley leaves
    c. 2 garlic cloves
    d. 1/2 teaspoon red chili flakes
    e. 1/4 cup olive oil
    f. 2 tablespoons red wine vinegar
    g. Salt to taste
- **Instructions**:
    h. Blend all ingredients in a food processor until smooth.
    i. Use as a sauce for grilled meats, fish, or roasted vegetables.

6. Polynesian Breadfruit Salad with Noni Dressing (Hawaii)
- **Benefits**: Supports immune health and regulates blood sugar.
- **Ingredients**:
    a. 1 medium breadfruit, boiled and cubed
    b. 1/2 cup diced pineapple
    c. 1/4 cup red onion, thinly sliced
    d. 1/4 cup noni juice
    e. 2 tablespoons coconut cream
    f. Salt and pepper to taste
- **Instructions**:
    g. Toss breadfruit, pineapple, and red onion in a large bowl.
    h. Whisk noni juice and coconut cream together, then pour over the salad.
    i. Season with salt and pepper and serve chilled.

Tips for Cooking with Medicinal Herbs
1. Fresh vs. Dried: Use fresh herbs for vibrant flavors and dried herbs for concentrated medicinal benefits.
2. Balance Flavors: Pair strong medicinal herbs with complementary ingredients to avoid overpowering the dish.
3. Low Heat: Cook herbs gently to preserve their active compounds.
4. Experiment: Add herbs to smoothies, soups, or baked goods to explore their versatility.

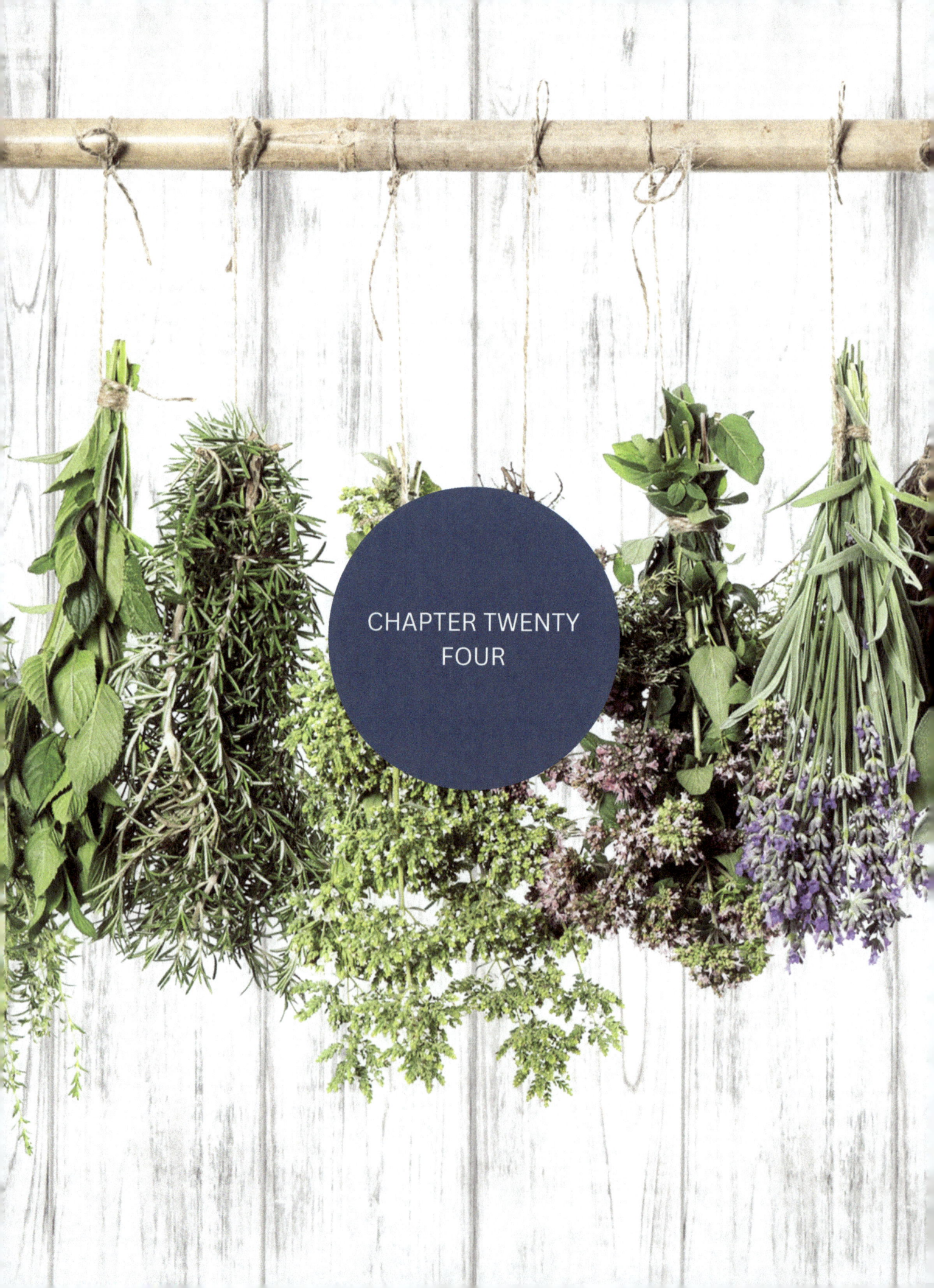

CHAPTER TWENTY FOUR

Seasonal Wellness with Herbs

The changing seasons bring unique health challenges, from colds and flu in the winter to allergies in the spring. Herbal remedies can provide natural, effective support to help the body adapt to these transitions. This chapter explores how to prepare for seasonal shifts with specific herbs, creating remedies that boost immunity, soothe allergies, and maintain overall health.

Preparing for Flu Season

Flu season often arrives with cold weather, and boosting the immune system beforehand can reduce the risk of illness. Herbal remedies can help protect the body and alleviate symptoms if sickness occurs.

Key Herbs for Flu Prevention and Relief

1. **Elderberry:** Strengthens the immune system and shortens the duration of colds and flu.
    - Recipe: Elderberry Syrup
        - Ingredients: 1 cup dried elderberries, 4 cups water, 1 cup honey.
        - Instructions: Simmer elderberries in water until reduced by half, strain, and mix with honey. Take 1 teaspoon daily.
2. **Echinacea:** Activates the immune system to ward off infections.
    - Use: Brew as tea or take as a tincture at the onset of symptoms.
3. **Ginger:** Relieves congestion and soothes sore throats.
    - Recipe: Ginger and Lemon Tea
        - Ingredients: 1-inch ginger root (sliced), juice of half a lemon, 1 teaspoon honey.
        - Instructions: Steep ginger in boiling water for 10 minutes, add lemon juice and honey, and sip warm.

Managing Allergy Season

Spring and early summer often bring allergies, with symptoms like sneezing, watery eyes, and congestion. Herbal remedies can help reduce inflammation and support the body's natural defenses.

Key Herbs for Allergy Relief

1. Nettle: Acts as a natural antihistamine to reduce allergy symptoms.
   - Use: Drink as tea or take in capsule form daily during allergy season.
2. Butterbur: Reduces nasal congestion and inflammation.
   - Use: Take as a standardized extract for maximum effectiveness.
3. Quercetin-Rich Herbs (e.g., Onion and Parsley): Stabilize mast cells to prevent histamine release.
   - Use: Incorporate into meals or take as a supplement.

Recipe: Allergy-Relief Tea

- Ingredients:
  - 1 teaspoon dried nettle leaves
  - 1 teaspoon chamomile
  - 1/2 teaspoon dried peppermint
  - Honey (optional)
- Instructions: Steep herbs in hot water for 5 minutes, strain, and enjoy twice daily.

Adapting to Seasonal Stressors

Each season presents unique stressors, from summer heat to winter fatigue. Herbs can help the body adapt to these changes and maintain energy and vitality.

For Winter Fatigue

- Ginseng: Boosts energy and stamina during colder months.
- Recipe: Ginseng Hot Chocolate
    - Ingredients: 1/2 teaspoon powdered ginseng, 1 cup hot milk (or plant-based alternative), 1 tablespoon cocoa powder, honey to taste.
    - Instructions: Stir all ingredients together and enjoy warm.

For Summer Heat

- Peppermint: Cools the body and soothes digestion.
- Recipe: Mint Cooler
    - Ingredients: Fresh mint leaves, 1 cup chilled water, juice of half a lime, honey to taste.
    - Instructions: Blend and serve over ice.

Year-Round Wellness Practices with Herbs
1. Adaptogens for All Seasons: Herbs like holy basil, ashwagandha, and reishi mushroom can help balance stress levels year-round.
2. Seasonal Detox: Incorporate dandelion and milk thistle to cleanse the liver and prepare the body for seasonal transitions.

By tailoring your herbal remedies to each season, you can support your body's natural rhythms and stay well throughout the year. These practices draw on the wisdom of herbal traditions to provide simple, natural solutions for seasonal wellness.

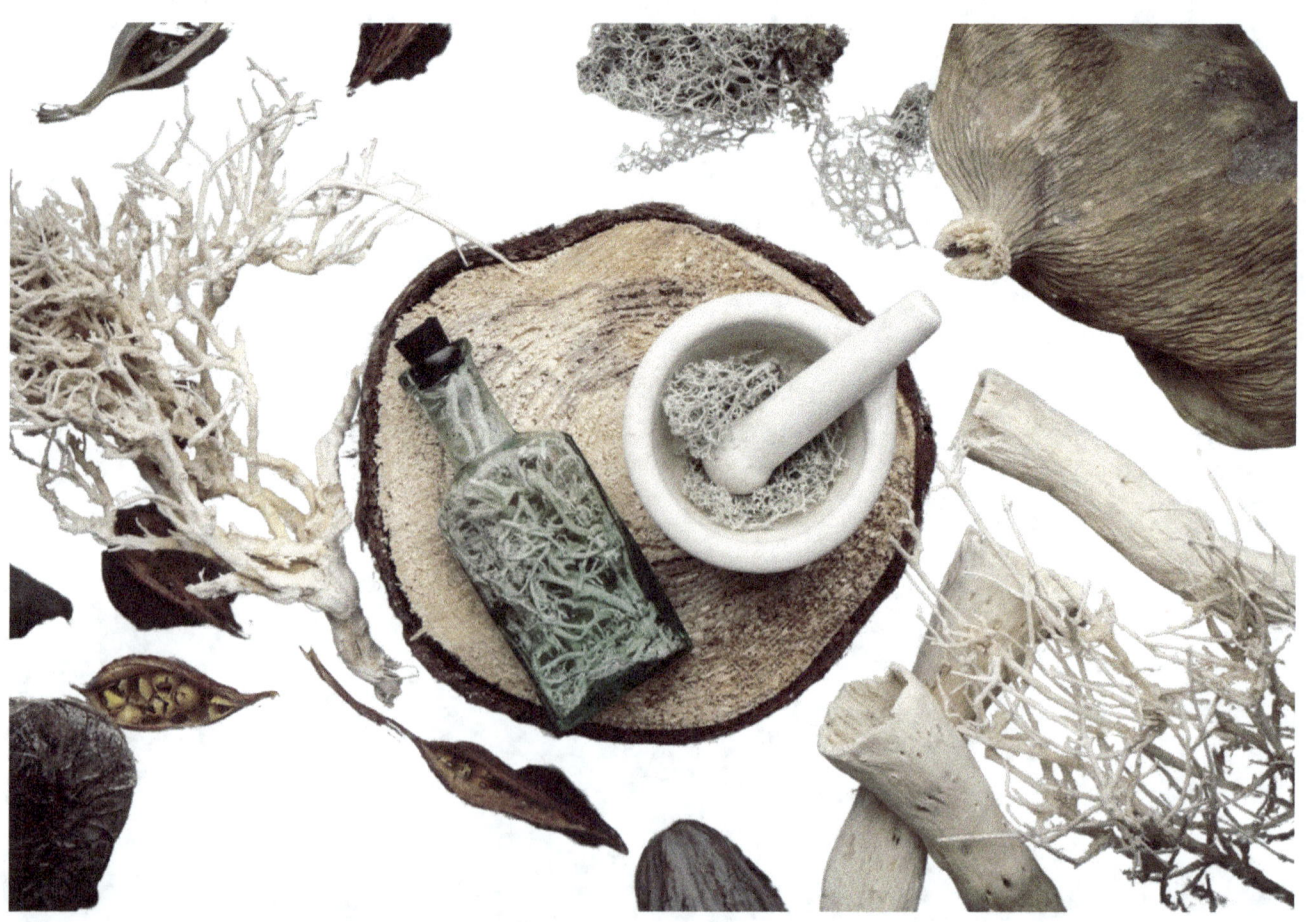

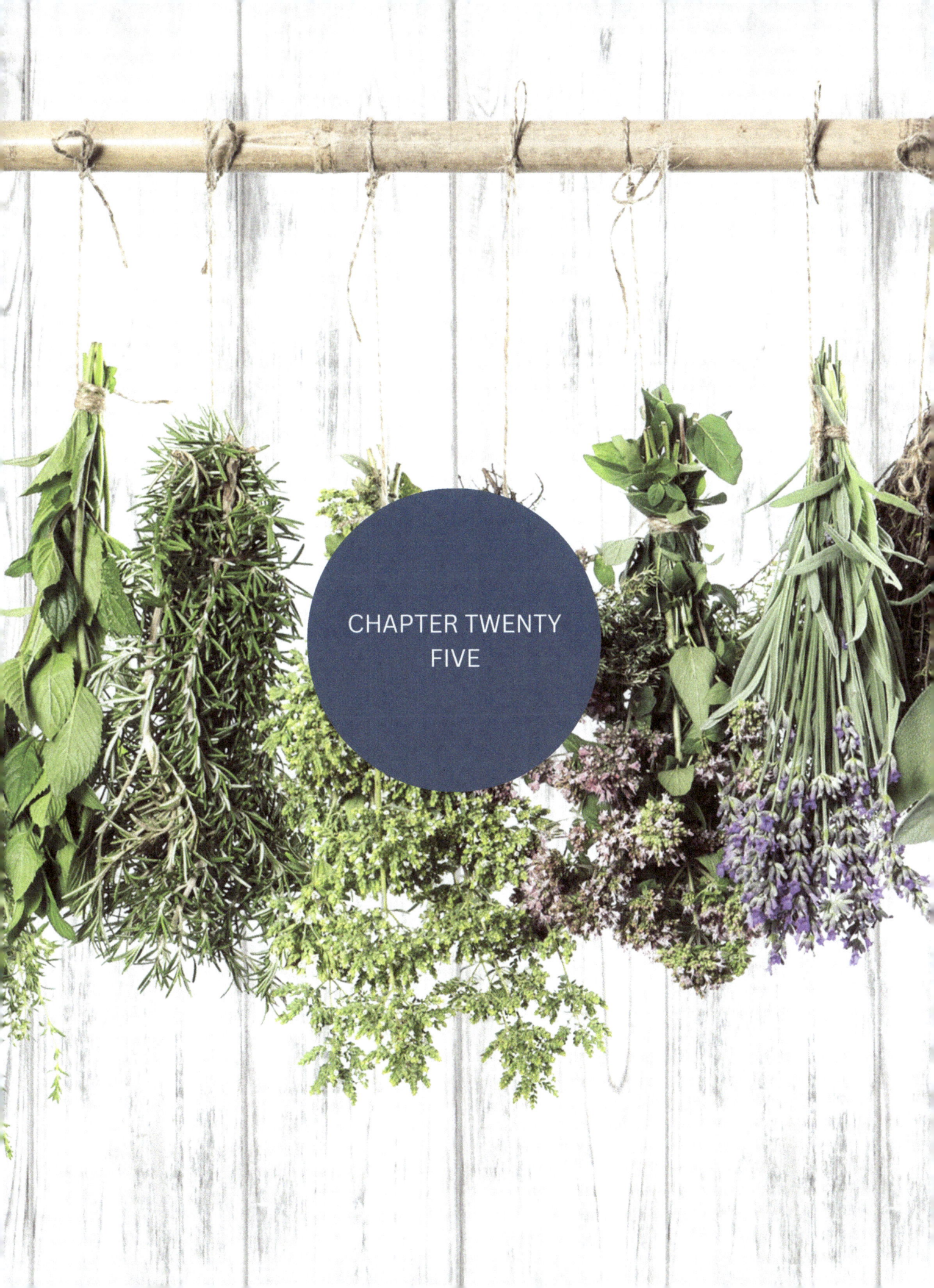

CHAPTER TWENTY FIVE

Herb Gardening Across Climates

Cultivating your herb garden allows you to have a fresh supply of medicinal and culinary herbs year-round. With careful planning, herbs from diverse climates—African, Asian, and European—can thrive at home, regardless of where you live. This chapter explores the essentials of herb gardening, from understanding climate needs to practical techniques for growing herbs indoors or outdoors.

Understanding Herb Climate Requirements

Each herb originates from specific climates, and replicating those conditions is key to their growth:

- African Herbs: Thrive in warm, sunny climates with well-drained soil. Examples include moringa, baobab, and hibiscus.
- Asian Herbs: Adaptable to tropical or temperate conditions, such as turmeric, ginseng, and holy basil (tulsi).
- European Herbs: Prefer cooler climates with moderate sunlight, such as lavender, chamomile, and thyme.

Preparing Your Garden

Whether planting outdoors, in containers, or indoors, preparing the right environment ensures healthy herbs:

1. Soil:
    - African Herbs: Sandy, well-drained soil enriched with organic matter.
    - Asian Herbs: Loamy soil with good moisture retention.

European Herbs: Light, slightly alkaline soil with adequate drainage.

1. **Sunlight**:
    - African herbs: 6–8 hours of full sun daily.
    - Asian herbs: Partial shade to full sun, depending on the plant.
    - European herbs: 4–6 hours of sunlight; some tolerate shade.
2. **Watering**:
    - African and Asian herbs often tolerate drought once established but require consistent watering initially.
    - European herbs prefer moderate watering—too much water can lead to root rot.

Growing African Herbs
1. **Moringa**:
    - **Climate**: Warm, arid regions.
    - **Planting**: Direct sow seeds in sandy soil; requires full sun.
    - **Care**: Water sparingly; prune regularly to encourage bushy growth.
2. **Hibiscus**:
    - **Climate**: Tropical to subtropical.
    - **Planting**: Propagate via cuttings or seeds in loamy soil.
    - **Care**: Water consistently; thrives in humid conditions.
3. **Neem**:
    - **Climate**: Hot, sunny regions.
    - **Planting**: Grows well from seeds or saplings.
    - **Care**: Needs full sun; minimal watering once established.

Growing Asian Herbs

1. Turmeric:
   - Climate: Warm, humid regions.
   - Planting: Plant rhizomes in pots or garden beds with rich, moist soil.
   - Care: Water regularly; harvest rhizomes after 8–10 months.
2. Holy Basil (Tulsi):
   - Climate: Tropical to subtropical.
   - Planting: Sow seeds in well-drained soil; requires full sun.
   - Care: Water lightly; pinch off flowers to prolong leaf production.
3. Ginseng:
   - Climate: Cool, shaded environments.
   - Planting: Prefers raised beds with rich, well-drained soil.

Care: Requires patience; takes 3–5 years to mature.

Growing European Herbs
1. Lavender:
    - Climate: Mediterranean, with warm summers and mild winters.
    - Planting: Grow in pots or garden beds with sandy, alkaline soil.
    - Care: Requires full sun; water sparingly.
2. Thyme:
    - Climate: Temperate, with good sunlight.
    - Planting: Sow seeds or use cuttings in well-drained soil.
    - Care: Water sparingly; thrives in dry conditions.
3. Chamomile:
    - Climate: Cool, moderate regions.
    - Planting: Direct sow seeds in light, well-drained soil.
    - Care: Needs partial sunlight; water moderately.

Herb Gardening Tips Across Climates

1. Indoor Herb Gardening:
     - Use pots with good drainage.
     - Place near a sunny window or use grow lights.
2. Seasonal Adjustments:
     - Protect tropical herbs from frost in winter by bringing pots indoors.
     - Mulch around temperate herbs to retain moisture during dry seasons.
3. Companion Planting:
     - Combine herbs with similar water and sunlight needs in the same bed or container.
4. Pest Control:
     - Use neem oil or garlic sprays as natural deterrents.

Global Gardening Challenges and Solutions
- Limited Space: Use vertical gardening or grow herbs in stacked pots.
- Harsh Climates: Modify conditions with greenhouses or shade cloths.
- Soil Issues: Improve with organic compost or pH adjustments.

By understanding the specific needs of African, Asian, and European herbs, gardeners can cultivate a diverse and thriving herb collection at home, unlocking the healing power of plants from around the world.

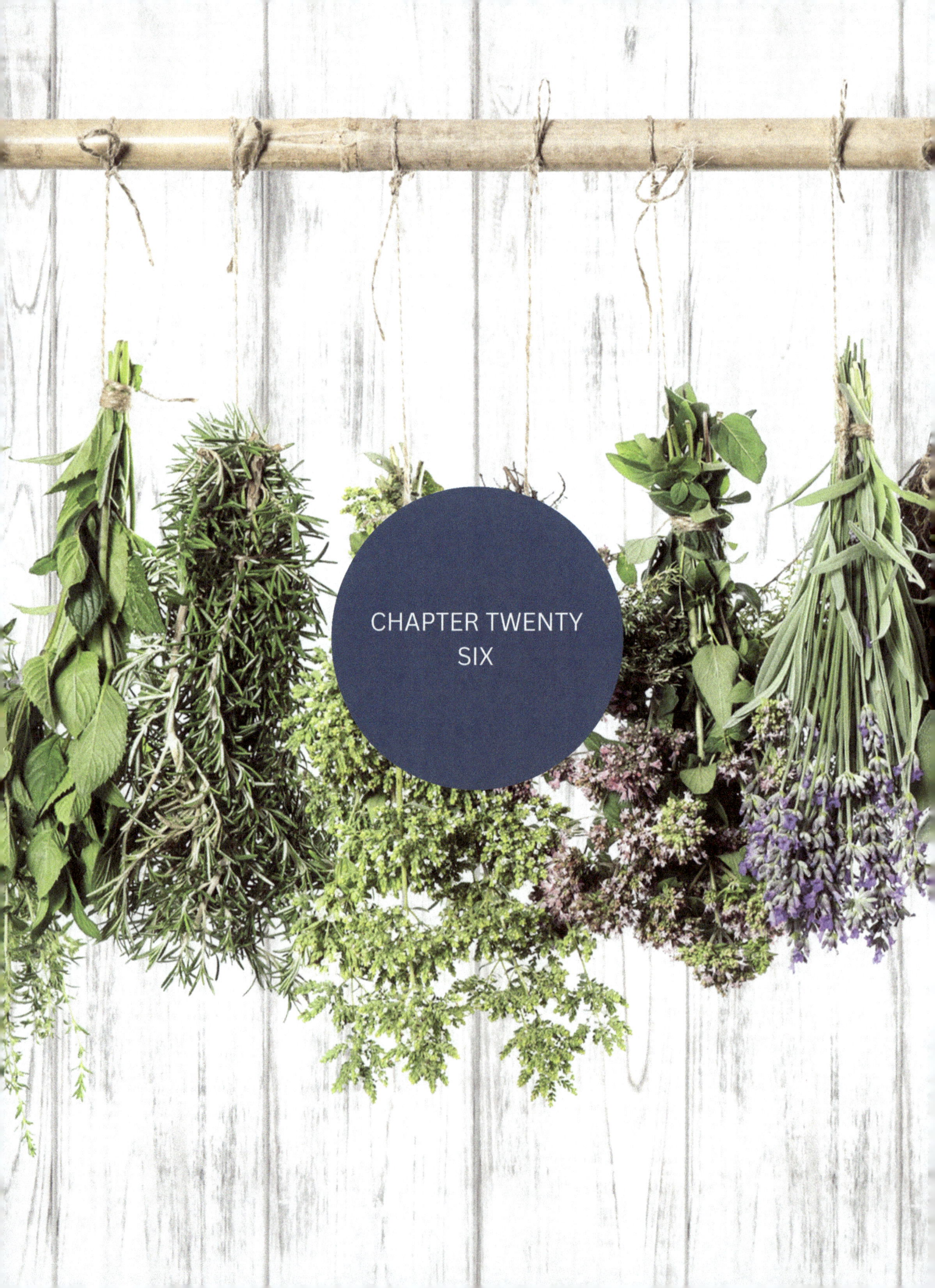

CHAPTER TWENTY SIX

Foraging and Ethical Harvesting

Foraging is the ancient practice of gathering wild herbs, plants, and natural resources directly from the environment. While foraging can be a rewarding and sustainable way to connect with nature and obtain herbs, it is crucial to approach it responsibly. Ethical harvesting ensures the preservation of ecosystems, protects endangered species, and respects cultural and community practices tied to the land.

Understanding Foraging

1. What Is Foraging?
   - The act of identifying, collecting, and using wild plants for food, medicine, or other purposes.
   - A practice deeply rooted in traditional cultures across the globe.
2. Why Forage?
   - Access to herbs in their natural, unaltered state.
   - Free, sustainable resource for herbal remedies.
   - Opportunity to reconnect with nature and develop plant identification skills.

Preparation for Ethical Foraging

1. Learn the Landscape:
   - Research Local Flora: Study native plants and their uses. Consult field guides or local experts.
   - Understand Ecosystems: Know which plants are abundant and which are endangered.
   - Know the Laws: Many areas have regulations about wild plant harvesting; ensure you have permission.
2. Identify Plants Correctly:
   - Use Guides: Bring a detailed plant identification book or app.
   - Learn from Experts: Join local foraging workshops or walks.

Double-Check: Misidentifying plants can be dangerous; some wild herbs have toxic look-alikes.

1. **Foraging Tools**:
   - **Cutting Tools**: Sharp scissors or pruning shears to minimize damage to plants.
   - **Containers**: Use baskets or breathable bags to keep herbs fresh.
   - **Notebook**: Record plant locations and notes for future reference.

Principles of Ethical Harvesting
1. **Harvest Sustainably**:
   - Take only what you need to allow plants to regenerate. A common rule is to harvest no more than 10% of the plant population in any area.
   - Avoid uprooting entire plants unless they are abundant and intended for transplant or propagation.
2. **Protect Endangered Species**:
   - Familiarize yourself with local endangered plants. Some herbs, like certain wild orchids, are rare and should not be foraged.
   - Substitute cultivated versions of rare plants whenever possible.
3. **Respect the Environment**:
   - Stay on trails to minimize habitat disruption.
   - Avoid foraging in polluted or contaminated areas, such as near roads or industrial zones.
4. **Respect Cultural and Local Practices**:
   - Be aware of traditional ownership or cultural significance attached to certain plants.
   - Seek permission when foraging on private or community land.

How to Harvest Herbs Responsibly
1. Leaves and Stems:
    - Harvest in the early morning when essential oils are most concentrated.
    - Snip leaves or stems from the middle or top, leaving the base to regrow.
2. Flowers:
    - Collect during peak bloom, ensuring pollinators have visited the plant.
    - Take only a few flowers from each plant.
3. Roots:
    - Dig carefully to avoid damaging surrounding plants.
    - Harvest mature plants and leave smaller ones to grow.
4. Seeds:
    - Allow seeds to mature fully before harvesting.
    - Leave enough seeds behind to ensure natural reproduction.
5. Bark:
    - Harvest only from mature trees, and never strip bark entirely around the trunk (this can kill the tree).
    - Use a small section from branches instead.

Post-Harvest Practices

1. Processing:
   - Wash herbs gently to remove dirt and insects.
   - Dry them in a cool, dark, and airy place to preserve potency.
2. Storing:
   - Use airtight containers to store dried herbs.
   - Label with the date and location of harvest to monitor freshness.
3. Giving Back:
   - Scatter seeds or plant saplings to replenish the ecosystem.
   - Support conservation initiatives and educate others on sustainable foraging.

Global Examples of Ethical Foraging

- African Context: Indigenous communities sustainably harvest baobab and moringa while preserving biodiversity in savannas.
- Asian Context: Traditional Chinese Medicine practices include controlled harvesting of herbs like ginseng to prevent overexploitation.
- European Context: Foragers in the UK and Scandinavia follow "right to roam" laws while adhering to strict harvesting guidelines to protect wild flora.
- North American Context: Native American traditions often involve ceremonies to honor the spirit of the plants being harvested.

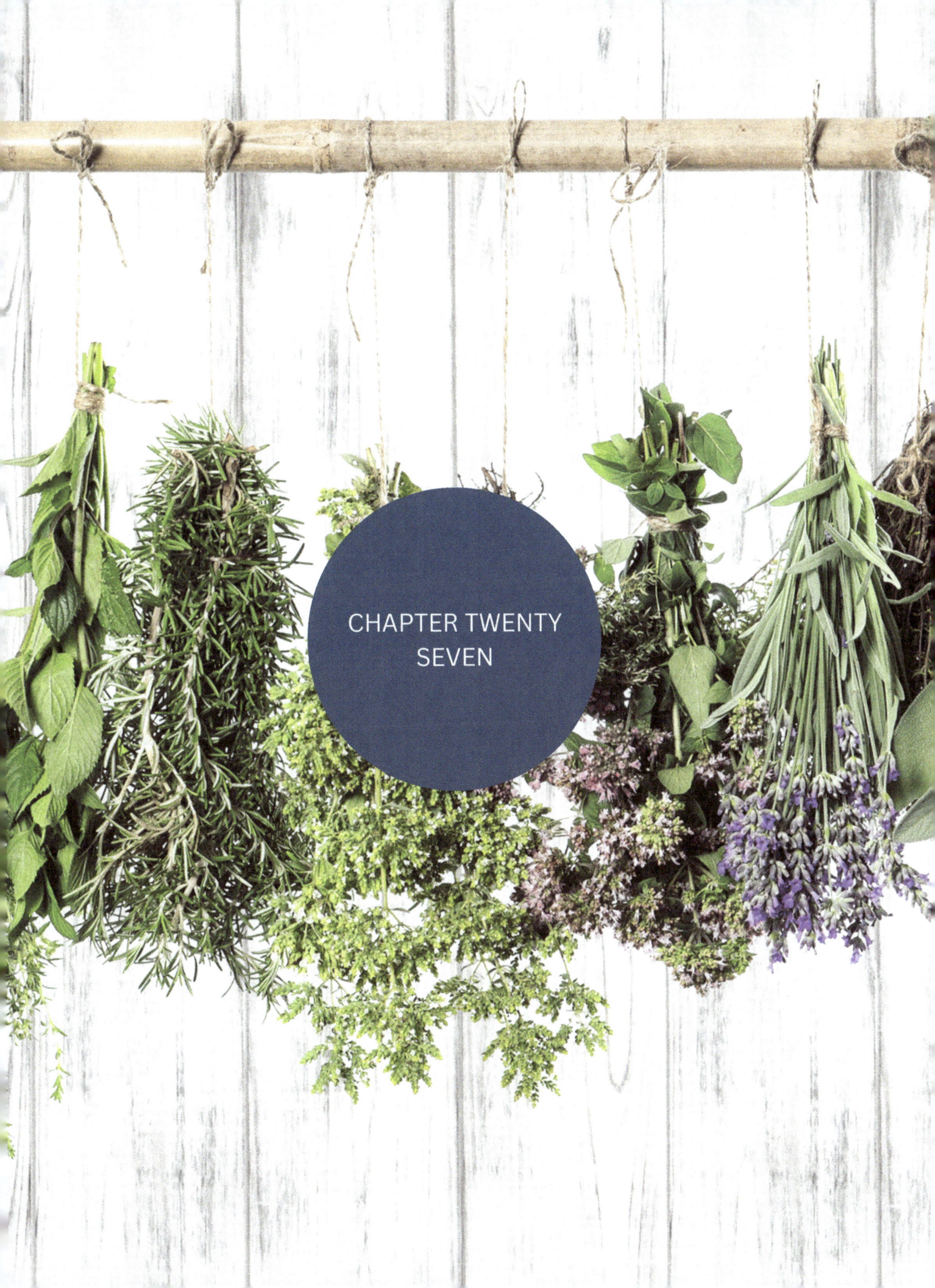

CHAPTER TWENTY SEVEN

Storing and Maintaining Your Remedies

Proper storage and maintenance of herbal remedies are critical to preserving their potency, effectiveness, and safety. Herbal products can lose their therapeutic value over time if exposed to heat, light, moisture, or air. This chapter explores methods to extend the shelf life of herbal preparations and maintain their quality.

Factors Affecting the Shelf Life of Herbal Remedies
1. Environmental Conditions:
    - Light: Direct sunlight can degrade active compounds in herbs, especially essential oils and tinctures.
    - Heat: High temperatures accelerate the breakdown of herbal components.
    - Moisture: Promotes mold and bacterial growth, especially in dried herbs.
    - Air: Exposure to oxygen can oxidize sensitive compounds, reducing potency.
2. Type of Preparation:
    - Dried Herbs: Have a longer shelf life when properly stored, typically 1–2 years.
    - Tinctures: Alcohol-based tinctures can last 5–10 years if stored correctly.
    - Oils and Salves: May last up to a year but are prone to rancidity if not kept in a cool, dark place.
    - Teas and Infusions: Best consumed within 24–48 hours to avoid microbial growth.
3. Quality of Ingredients:
    - Fresh, high-quality herbs result in remedies with a longer shelf life and better effectiveness.
    - Always use clean, sterilized tools and containers to prevent contamination.

Storage Techniques for Herbal Remedies

1. Dried Herbs:
   - Store in airtight containers, such as glass jars with tight-fitting lids.
   - Use dark-colored jars or store in a dark cupboard to minimize light exposure.
   - Add silica gel packets to control moisture in the storage area.
   - Label with the date of drying and source to track freshness.
2. Tinctures:
   - Use dark amber or cobalt glass bottles to protect against light.
   - Store in a cool, dry place, such as a pantry or cupboard.
   - Label with the date of preparation and the herb used.
3. Herbal Oils and Salves:
   - Keep in dark glass jars or tins to reduce light exposure.
   - Refrigeration can extend the shelf life of herbal oils prone to rancidity.
   - Use a clean spatula or spoon when handling to prevent contamination.
4. Teas, Infusions, and Decoctions:
   - Prepare only the quantity you intend to use within a day or two.
   - Store in the refrigerator in a covered container for up to 48 hours.
5. Capsules and Powders:
   - Store in airtight containers, away from heat and humidity.
   - Use silica gel packets in the container to prevent clumping from moisture.
6. Essential Oils:
   - Keep in tightly sealed dark glass bottles.
   - Store in a cool, dark place to prevent evaporation and degradation.

Extending the Shelf Life of Herbal Products
1. Use Preservatives:
    - For water-based remedies like creams, consider natural preservatives like vitamin E, rosemary extract, or grapefruit seed extract.
    - Alcohol in tinctures acts as a natural preservative.
2. Sterilize Equipment and Containers:
    - Clean and sterilize all jars, bottles, and tools before use to prevent bacterial or mold contamination.
3. Avoid Cross-Contamination:
    - Use clean utensils or hands when handling herbal products.
    - Keep remedies in tightly sealed containers to prevent exposure to airborne contaminants.
4. Monitor for Signs of Spoilage:
    - Check for changes in color, odor, or texture.
    - Discard any remedies that show signs of mold, rancidity, or an unusual smell.

Rotating and Managing Inventory
1. Labeling:
   - Always label remedies with preparation dates and expiration estimates.
   - Include information about the herb and preparation method for quick reference.
2. First In, First Out:
   - Use older remedies before newer batches to minimize waste.
   - Regularly inspect your inventory and discard expired products.
3. Regular Inspections:
   - Periodically check remedies for signs of spoilage or degradation.
   - Maintain a log to track which remedies are due for use or disposal.

Best Practices for Long-Term Storage
1. Freeze Dried Herbs:
   - Freeze drying is an excellent method for long-term preservation while maintaining potency.
   - Store freeze-dried herbs in vacuum-sealed bags or jars.
2. Vacuum Sealing:
   - For dried herbs, vacuum sealing removes air and extends shelf life.
   - Combine with refrigeration or freezing for optimal results.
3. Desiccant Use:
   - Place desiccant packets in storage containers to absorb residual moisture.
4. Dedicated Storage Area:
   - Create a designated space for your herbal products that is cool, dry, and dark.
   - Keep storage areas organized to prevent accidental damage or exposure.

Glossary of Herbs and Active Compounds

This section provides a concise reference for the key herbs and active compounds discussed in the book, helping readers identify their properties and benefits.

Glossary of Herbs

1. Moringa (Africa): Known as the "Miracle Tree," it is rich in vitamins, minerals, and antioxidants.
2. Ginseng (Asia): Boosts energy, improves concentration, and enhances immunity.
3. Lavender (Europe): A calming herb used for relaxation and skin care.
4. Echinacea (Native America): Stimulates the immune system and fights colds.
5. Kava (Polynesia): Reduces anxiety and promotes relaxation.

Glossary of Active Compounds

1. Curcumin: Found in turmeric; known for its potent anti-inflammatory and antioxidant properties.
2. Saponins: Present in plants like licorice root; beneficial for immune health and cholesterol management.
3. Alkaloids: Found in herbs such as black cohosh; offer pain-relieving and anti-inflammatory benefits.
4. Flavonoids: Common in chamomile and hibiscus; support heart health and reduce inflammation.
5. Tannins: Found in thyme and sage; have antimicrobial and astringent properties.

Index of Remedies by Ailment

Organized for ease of access, this index helps readers locate herbal remedies based on specific health concerns.

Immune Support
- Colds and Flu: Echinacea, Elderberry, Holy Basil
- Allergies: Nettle, Butterbur

Digestive Health
- Bloating and Gas: Peppermint, Fennel
- Nausea: Ginger, Chamomile

Stress and Mental Health
- Anxiety: Kava, Ashwagandha
- Cognitive Health: Gotu Kola, Ginseng

Skin Care
- Acne: Neem, Tea Tree Oil
- Wound Healing: Yarrow, Aloe Vera

Chronic Pain
- Joint Pain: Devil's Claw, Willow Bark
- Muscle Pain: Arnica, St. John's Wort

Suggested Further Reading and Courses

Enhance your knowledge of herbal medicine with these curated books, articles, and educational programs.

Books
1. The Complete Guide to Medicinal Herbs by Penelope Ody
2. Adaptogens: Herbs for Strength, Stamina, and Stress Relief by David Winston
3. Herbal Medicine: From the Heart of the Earth by Sharol Tilgner

Articles and Journals
1. "Herbal Therapeutics: The Science Behind the Tradition" (Journal of Herbal Medicine)
2. "Ethnobotany and Its Applications" (Nature Reviews Drug Discovery)

Online Courses
1. Herbal Academy: Foundations of Herbal Medicine Certificate Program
2. American Botanical Council: Herbal Research and Educational Webinars
3. Coursera: Herbal Medicine and Holistic Health Practices

Final Note

As you close the pages of The Homemade Apothecary, I hope you carry with you a renewed sense of empowerment and connection to the natural world. This book is more than a guide; it is an invitation to rediscover the healing power of herbs, to embrace sustainable and holistic living, and to cherish the wisdom passed down through generations across the globe.

Herbal medicine is as much about the journey as it is about the destination. Every herb you grow, every remedy you craft, and every moment you spend in harmony with nature deepens your understanding of the delicate balance between our well-being and the world around us.

Remember, the knowledge you've gained here is not static. It grows with your curiosity, your experiences, and your willingness to learn. Share what you've discovered with others, pass on traditions, and inspire those around you to explore the beauty of natural healing.

Whether you're addressing a personal health concern, nurturing a loved one, or simply seeking a moment of peace in your daily life, let this book serve as your trusted companion. Keep exploring, keep experimenting, and, most importantly, keep healing—mind, body, and soul.

Thank you for allowing me to be part of your herbal journey. May your home apothecary flourish, bringing health, joy, and harmony to your life.

With heartfelt gratitude,

Maggie Damien, PhD

www.ingramcontent.com/pod-product-compliance
Lightning Source LLC
Chambersburg PA
CBHW062214220526
45471CB00009B/3202